CRANIOFACIAL PROSTHESES
ANAPLASTOLOGY AND OSSEOINTEGRATION

CRANIOFACIAL PROSTHESES
ANAPLASTOLOGY AND OSSEOINTEGRATION

Edited by

PER-INGVAR BRÅNEMARK, MD, PHD

Professor and Director
Institute for Applied Biotechnology
Gothenburg, Sweden

MARCELO FERRAZ DE OLIVEIRA, DDS

Maxillofacial Prosthodontist
Institute for Applied Biotechnology
Gothenburg, Sweden

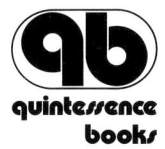

Quintessence Publishing Co, Inc
Chicago, Berlin, London, Tokyo, Paris, Barcelona, São Paulo, Moscow, Prague, and Warsaw

Pictures of the replica of Greek sculpture from the Antique Museum in Lund, Sweden, were provided by:
Eva Strömvall, photographer (Atelje Bjerred)
Anne-Marie Leander-Touati, Department of Classical Studies,
University of Lund
Jan Hellberg, hand model
Kajsa Wipp, graphic designer

Library of Congress Cataloging-in-Publication Data
Craniofacial prostheses: anaplastology and osseointegration/edited by Per-Ingvar Brånemark,
  Marcelo Ferraz de Oliveira.
     p.   cm.
  Includes bibliographical references.
  ISBN 0-86715-321-0
  1. Head—Surgery. 2. Prosthesis. 3. Surgery, Plastic. 4. Osseointegration. 5. Maxillofacial prosthesis.
  6. Ear prostheses.   I. Brånemark, Per-Ingvar. II. Oliveira, Marcelo Ferraz de.
     [DNLM: 1. Maxillofacial Prosthesis. 2. Osseointegration. 3. Ear, External 4. Nose. 5. Surgery, Plastic—
     methods. 6. Neoplasms—complications. WU 600 C891 1997]
RD521.C73 1997
617.5'10592–dc21
DNLM/DLC
for Library of Congress   96–50068
                                                                    CIP

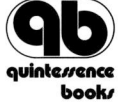

©1997 by Quintessence Publishing Co, Inc

Published by Quintessence Publishing Co, Inc
551 N. Kimberly Drive
Carol Stream, IL 60188

All rights reserved. This book or any part thereof may not be reproduced, stored in a retrieval system,
or transmitted in any form or by any means, electronic, mechanical, photocopying, recording, or
otherwise, without prior written permission of the publisher.

Editor: Patricia Bereck Weikersheimer
Assistant Editor: Lane Evensen
Designer: Jennifer A. Sabella
Printed in Hong Kong

Contents

Contributors   vii
Preface   ix

Part I
Anaplastology: The Art of Prosthetic Reconstruction

Introduction   3
  Ann Fyler

Acknowledgments   5

Key to Clinicians   8

Patient Presentations   9
  Auricular Defects   11
  Nasal Defects   37
  Orbital Defects   49
  Complex Defects   67

Part II
Osseointegration: Anchorage of Craniofacial Prostheses

Introduction   85
  P-I Brånemark

1 Craniomaxillofacial Rehabilitation in Oncology Patients   86
   Philip Worthington

2 Plastic and Reconstructive Surgery   92
   Elof Eriksson

3 Opportunity for Maxillofacial Prosthetics   96
   Patrick Henry

4 Anaplastological Technique for Facial Defects   101
   Kerstin Bergström

5 IMPAIRED FUNCTION OF THE TEMPOROMANDIBULAR JOINT IN ONCOLOGY PATIENTS   111
   Ragnar Adell

6 HYPERBARIC OXYGEN TREATMENT OF FORMER CANCER PATIENTS TO SUPPORT OSSEOINTEGRATION   115
   Gösta Granström

7 PSYCHOLOGICAL CONSIDERATIONS IN THE TREATMENT OF PATIENTS WITH CANCER   118
   Stig Blomberg

8 FACIAL RECONSTRUCTION FOLLOWING CANCER TREATMENT: A CASE STUDY   120
   Elaine Williams

CONCLUDING REMARKS   125
   P-I Brånemark

Contributors

Ragnar Adell, DDS, PhD
Associate Professor and Head
Department of Oral and Maxillofacial
 Surgery
Örebro Medical Center Hospital
Örebro, Sweden

Kerstin Bergström, CDT, MDhc
Anaplastologist
Department of Otolaryngology
Sahlgren's University Hospital
University of Gothenburg
Gothenburg, Sweden

Stig Blomberg, MD, PhD
Associate Professor
Department of Psychiatry
University of Gothenburg
Mölndal, Sweden

Per-Ingvar Brånemark, MD, PhD
Professor
Institute for Applied Biotechnology
Gothenburg, Sweden

Julie Jordan Brown, MAMS
Anaplastologist/Certified Medical
 Illustrator
Medical Art Resources, Inc.
Milwaukee, Wisconsin

Enrique de Damborenea
Maxillofacial Technologist/
 Anaplastologist
Madrid, Spain

Gillian F. Duncan, MS
Medical Illustrator/Anaplastologist
Institute for Epitheses
Graphica-Sculptura Medica
Rochester, Minnesota

Elof Eriksson, MD
Professor and Chief of Plastic Surgery
Department of Surgery
Harvard Medical School
Boston, Massachusetts

Peter Evans, MIMPT
Chief Maxillofacial Prosthetist
Maxillofacial Unit
Welsh Centre for Burns, Plastic and
 Maxillofacial Surgery
Morriston Hospital
Swansea, Wales

Ann Fyler, BS
Medical Artist/Anaplastologist
Director, Clinic of Anaplastology
Department of Otolaryngology
University of Iowa Hospitals and
 Clinics
Iowa City, Iowa

Gregory G. Gion, BS
Medical Artist/Anaplastologist
Maxillofacial and Somato Prosthetics
Dallas, Texas

Gösta Granström, MD, DDS, PhD
Associate Professor
Department of E.N.T. Surgery
Sahlgren's University Hospital
University of Gothenburg
Gothenburg, Sweden

Steven J. Gray
Clinical Anaplastologist
Manager, Anaplastology Department
 and Brånemark Implant Program
Plastic and Reconstructive Surgery
 Unit
Alfred Hospital
Melbourne, Australia

Susan Habakuk, MEd
Medical Artist/Anaplastologist
Maxillofacial Prosthetics Clinic
The Craniofacial Center
College of Medicine
University of Illinois
Chicago, Illinois

Irene Healey, AOCA, BScAAM
Medical Artist/Anaplastologist
Process Coordinator
Craniofacial Prosthetics Unit
Toronto Sunnybrook Regional Cancer
 Centre
Toronto, Canada

Patrick J. Henry, DDS
Director
The Brånemark Osseointegration
 Center
West Perth, Western Australia

Iain Mathieson, MIMPT
Senior Chief Maxillofacial Prosthetist
 and Technologist
Crosshouse Hospital
Kilmarnock, Ayrshire
Scotland

David C. Mcnamara, BDSc, MDSc, PhD
Prosthodontist
Plastic and Maxillofacial Surgery Unit
Royal Perth Hospital
Perth, Australia

Lou Ann Mercier, MAMS
Medical Artist/Anaplastologist
Division of Anaplastology
Department of Otolaryngology
University of Iowa Hospitals and
 Clinics
Iowa City, Iowa

Marcelo Ferraz de Oliveira, DDS
Maxillofacial Prosthodontist
Institute for Applied Biotechnology
Gothenburg, Sweden

Ann-Marie Riedinger-Keller, MA
Medical Artist/Anaplastologist
Niederhausbergen, France

Paula J. Sauerborn, BFA
Director, Center for Prosthetic
 Restorations, Inc
Baltimore, Maryland

Keith Thomas, FIMPT
Clinical Prosthetist
Prosthesis and Camouflage Clinic
St. Andrews Centre for Plastic Surgery
St. Andrews Hospital
Billericay, Essex
England

David Trainer, LGCI
Facial Prosthetist
Institute for Epitheses Strunk
Siegen-Gosenbach, Germany

Elaine Williams, BSc
Kent, England

Johan Wolfaardt, BDS, MDent, PhD
Craniofacial Osseointegration and
 Maxillofacial Prosthetic
 Rehabilitation Unit
Misericordia Hospital
Faculty of Medicine and Oral Health
 Sciences
University of Alberta
Edmonton, Canada

Steve Worrollo, MIMPT
Maxillofacial Prosthetist
University Hospital Birmingham
NHS Trust
Queen Elizabeth Hospital
Birmingham, England

Philip Worthington, MD
Professor and Chairman
Department of Oral and Maxillofacial
 Surgery
School of Dentistry
University of Washington
Seattle, Washington

Preface

CONGENITAL OR TRAUMATIC LOSS of minor or major parts of head and neck anatomy requires reconstruction with biologic or synthetic substitutes. This is particularly demanding after radical resection of tumors.

This book is composed of two parts in order to emphasize the two decisive components in prosthetic craniomaxillofacial rehabilitation.

Anaplastology is a basic prerequisite for rehabilitation, providing a prosthetic substitute for lost anatomy that looks normal, both topographically and optically, and has borders that become part of the movements of the adjacent tissue. Considerable skill and experience is required to create such a prosthesis.

Osseointegrated stability in the connector of the prosthesis to the defect region is another important requirement for rehabilitation. The principle of osseointegration has had long-term successful application in anchoring artificial substitutes for teeth. This has prompted development of modified hardware and software for use in reconstruction of even major maxillofacial defects. Osseointegration makes it possible to stabilize a prosthesis in a reliable and predictable manner.

Because of the often compromised local tissues, careful planning and performance of the surgical procedures are required. In addition, the often complex psychosocial consequences of minor and major craniomaxillofacial defects need special attention and necessitate a team approach for successful results.

In Part I of this book, a series of examples are given, from different parts of the world, of what can be provided by anaplastologists irrespective of how the prosthesis is connected to the patient (whether by adhesive; by retention, designing the base of the prosthesis to extend into anatomical cavities; or by direct anchorage into bone tissue).

In Part II, representatives of specialties involved share their experience and advice on how to optimize treatment planning and the overall results of prosthetic rehabilitation.

Part I
Anaplastology: The Art of Prosthetic Reconstruction

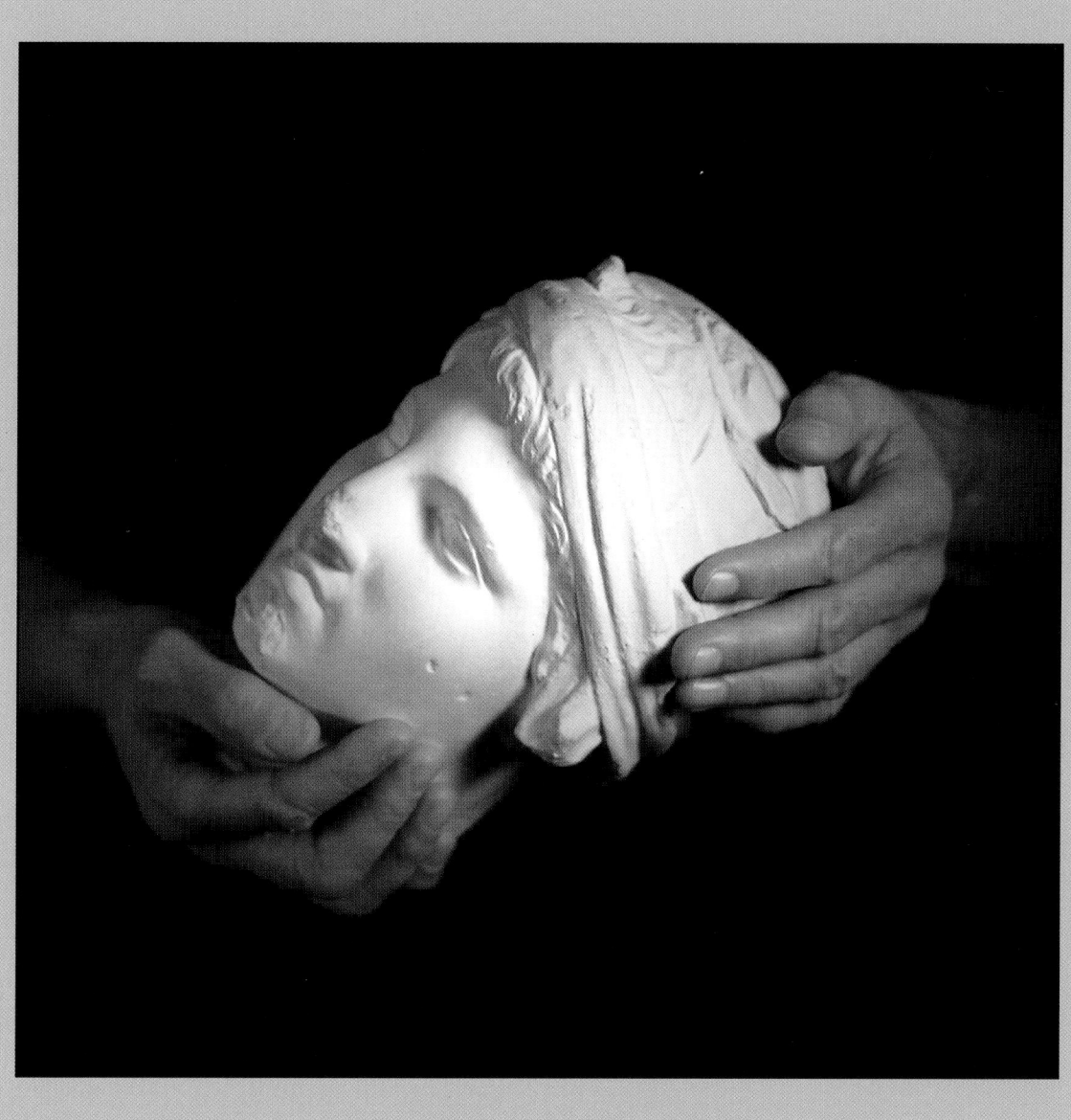

Introduction

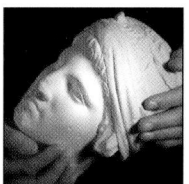

Ann Fyler

ANAPLASTOLOGY IS THE ART AND SCIENCE of restoring malformed or absent parts of the face or body by artificial means. It provides prosthetic restoration, external to the oral cavity, for patients with disfigurements from disease, trauma, or congenital anomalies. Practitioners in the field of anaplastology come from a number of related disciplines. Its broad definition acknowledges the participation of medical, dental, artistic, and scientific professionals in providing prosthetic restorative care for patients and in advancing the knowledge of materials and techniques.

Anaplastology is, in a sense, an ancient craft surviving within the tertiary medical community in a high-tech world. To fabricate a prosthesis, artistic skills and sensibilities are necessary, first to perceive the form, texture, and colors present in the body; and then to replicate them so that the artificial part appears to be growing out of the body. The form sculpted of wax or clay must be anatomically accurate and personalized to the individual patient. It must yield thin, unnoticeable edges.

When the form is converted to silicone or other plastic materials, color is mixed to mimic even the smallest details of the histology of skin in its various layers. A study of light-mixing theory is necessary but not sufficient. Study of pigment mixing is also needed because each pigment is a chemical entity that, mixed with other pigments and a medium, creates a color dependent on the chemistry of the components. Colorants can be fugitive or stable, and each color palette must be learned by empirical experience. The crafts of sculpting and painting may be as old as humanity, but the fabrication of prostheses involves more. A thorough understanding of materials and technical processes, of the principles and practice of retention, of basic medical science, and of patients' health conditions and related multidisciplinary treatment planning is equally important.

Anaplastology is both driven and limited by current materials, technologies, and research. Some of the earliest prostheses, in the nineteenth century and before, were made of ivory or hammered copper (which was then painted) because these materials were available. Today, most facial and cosmetic limb prostheses are made of silicones, sometimes combined with other plastic or metal materials. Silicones offer ease of fabrication and color modification, resulting in prostheses that mimic intrinsic tissue coloration and the flexibility of cutaneous and muscular structures. But silicone does not have the self-cleansing, replicating, and repair properties of skin. It is subject to abrasion, tearing, yellowing, and the discoloration caused by absorption of environmental contaminants, such as smoke and body excretions. As a result, silicone prostheses need periodic replacement to maintain esthetics.

But even an esthetically perfect prosthesis, if not well retained, is as useless to the patient as a perfectly retained prosthesis in which poor esthetics draw attention to the defect. Optimal prosthetic retention relies on securing the prosthesis to fixed or stable tissues or a mechanical device. Where the defect is small and the supporting tissues are not very mobile (such as the bridge of the nose) conventional adhesive-retained prostheses may suffice. When the defect is large or the prosthesis could be dislodged by its projection or lack or adequate tissue support, a percutaneous osseointegrated-implant–retained prosthesis may be the treatment of choice. In any case, the anaplastologist must have an understanding of the anatomical and histological structures on which facial prostheses rest in order to design prostheses for optimal security under dynamic action. The anaplastologist who understands the interdependence of esthetics and retention will also appreciate the team approach needed for optimal prosthetic restoration.

Thus anaplastology functions within the larger medical community. Practitioners of anaplastology must maintain the same levels of ethics, professionalism, hygiene, and patient care as practitioners of medicine and dentistry. Cross-disciplinary communication is imperative, since patients needing prostheses are seen by numerous medical, surgical, and dental specialties. And since successful prosthetic restoration can depend on proper surgical preparation, presurgical consultation is crucial.

This book highlights what is possible now. The use of alloplastic materials in or on the body is here to stay. Medical science has taken great strides toward the early detection of cancer, thereby preventing the necessity of excavating huge areas of tissue. Advances in microvascular surgery allow closure of defects and the reattachment of amputated tissues formerly thought impossible. Material scientists may invent a flexible matrix through which myocutaneous tissue can grow, but a long time will pass before the globe of the eye will be replaced by transplant with functioning retinal innervation.

There exist today technologies that can measure the color reflectance of skin or fashion form via video/computer imaging and computer-controlled cutting machines. But even with the help of these technologies, the anaplastologist must still mix the colorants into the silicone or plastic medium and fit a form to a particular disfiguring defect, adjusting it to blend with the individual patient's overall features. This is the judgment and art that fits into the high-tech wrapping.

Acknowledgments

It is imperative to emphasize that the complexity of the forthcoming clinical cases required a multidisciplinary approach. The rehabilitation of these patients could not have been achieved without the cooperation of professionals from different specialties within the medical field. Thus, we want to thank all professionals involved in the rehabilitation of the patients presented and the institutions at which the procedures were performed:

Section I Auricular defects

1. Anders Tjellström, MD, PhD
   Gösta Granström, MD, DDS, PhD
   Sahlgren's University Hospital
   Gothenburg, Sweden

2. Mayo Clinic team
   Rochester, Minnesota

3. Adrian Sugar, MD
   Allan Bocca
   Morriston Hospital
   Swansea, Wales

4. Bonnie Hoffman
   University of Iowa
   Iowa City, Iowa

5. Veterans Affairs Medical Center
   Dallas, Texas

6. Pierre Sibille, MD
   Pierre Sabin, MD
   CHU de Nancy
   Denis Herman, MD
   CHU de Strasbourg
   France

7. Denis Herman, MD
   CHU de Strasbourg
   France

8. Anders Tjellström
   Sahlgren's University Hospital
   Gothenburg, Sweden

9. P. J. Weller
   St. Andrews Hospital
   Billericay, Essex
   England

10. Wolfgang Draf, MD
    Rainer Keerl, MD
    Clinic for Ear, Nose, and Throat
      Diseases and Plastic Facial Surgery
    Fulda City Clinics
    Fulda, Germany

11. Gordon Wilkes, MD
    Johan Wolfaardt, BDS
    Compru-Misericordia Hospital
    Edmonton, Canada

12. Michael J. Wake, MD
    David Proops, MD
    Queen Elizabeth Hospital
    Birmingham, England

13. Ralph Gilbert, MD
    Jim Anderson, BDS
    Sunnybrook Hospital
    Toronto, Canada

14. Barry Goldsmith, MD
    Michael Goldman, MD
    David Reisberg, DDS
    The Craniofacial Center
    University of Illinois
    Chicago, Illinois

15. Anders Tjellström
    Gösta Granström
    Sahlgren's University Hospital
    Gothenburg, Sweden

16. E. J. Anstee, MD
    Alfred Hospital
    Melbourne, Australia

17 Per-Ingvar Brånemark, MD
   E. J. Anstee, MD
   Alfred Hospital
   Melbourne, Australia

18 A. Baker, MD
   H. McComb, MD
   Patrick J. Henry, DDS
   Paul Barnsley
   Robert Mann
   Plastic and Maxillofacial Surgery
     Unit
   Royal Perth Hospital
   Perth, Australia

19 Raj Singh, MD, OBE
   Crosshouse Hospital
   Kilmarnock, Ayrshire
   Scotland

20 Graphica Medica
   Institute for Epitheses
   Hamburg/Saar, Germany

Section II Nasal defects

1 Michael Maves, MD
  Department of Otolaryngology
  University of Iowa
  Iowa City, Iowa

2 Henry Hoffman, MD
  Department of Otolaryngology
  University of Iowa
  Iowa City, Iowa

3 Henry Hoffman, MD
  Department of Otolaryngology
  University of Iowa
  Iowa City, Iowa

4 William Panje, MD
  Department of Otolaryngology
  University of Iowa
  Iowa City, Iowa

5 Tibor Ruff, MD
  H. Steve Byrd, MD
  Scott and White Hospital
  Temple, Texas
  Bruce Barbash, DDS
  Dallas, Texas

6 Dieter Housmann, MD
  Leverkusen, Germany

7 Ralph Gilbert, MD
  Jim Anderson, BDS
  Sunnybrook Hospital
  Toronto, Canada

8 William J. Moran, MD
  Eric Asher
  University of Illinois
  Chicago, Illinois

9 A. Baker, MD
  H. McComb, MD
  Patrick J. Henry, DDS
  Paul Barnsley
  Robert Mann
  Plastic and Maxillofacial Surgery
    Unit
  Royal Perth Hospital
  Perth, Australia

Section III Orbital defects

1 Anders Tjellström
  Gösta Granström
  Sahlgren's University Hospital
  Gothenburg, Sweden

2 J. R. Barton, MD
  Russell S. Gonnering, MD, SC
  Milwaukee, Wisconsin

3 Graphica Medica
  Institute for Epitheses
  Hamburg/Saar, Germany

4 Adrian Sugar, MD
  Allan Bocca
  Morriston Hospital
  Swansea, Wales

5 Per-Ingvar Brånemark, MD, PhD
  Kenji Higuchi, DDS, MS
  Michael Maves, MD
  Jeffrey Nered, MD
  William LaVelle, DDS, MS
  University of Iowa
  Iowa City, Iowa

6 David Tse, MD
  Bascom-Palmer Eye Institute
  Miami, Florida

7 David Sanders, MD
  Medical City Hospital
  Dallas, Texas

8 James Merritt, MD
   Medical City Hospital
   Dallas, Texas

9 Nicholas Iliff, MD
   Paul Manson, MD

10 D. K. Madan
   St. Andrews Hospital
   Billericay, Essex
   England

11 Dieter Housmann, MD
   Leverkusen, Germany

12 Andreas Bremerich, MD
   Clinic for Maxillofacial Surgery
   Bremen, Germany

13 Michael J. Wake, MD
   David Proops, MD
   Queen Elizabeth Hospital
   Birmingham, England

14 Henry Hoffman, MD
   Keith Carter, MD
   Department of Otolaryngology
   University of Iowa
   Iowa City, Iowa

15 Per-Ingvar Brånemark, MD
   M. K. Leung, MD
   H. Clelend, MD
   Alfred Hospital
   Melbourne, Australia

SECTION IV COMPLEX DEFECTS

1 John Frodel, MD
   Henry Hoffman, MD
   Dennis Crocket, MD
   Gary Funk, MD
   Kenneth Kempf, DDS
   Robert Novo, DDS
   Robert Olsen, DDS
   Kirk Fridrich, DDS
   Michael Arcuri, DDS
   Marcelo F. Oliveira, DDS
   University of Iowa
   Iowa City, Iowa

2 Per-Ingvar Brånemark, MD, PhD
   Kenji Higuchi, DDS, MS
   Antonio Assunção, MD
   Laércio Vasconcelos, DDS
   Carlos Eduardo Francischone, DDS
   Marcelo F. Oliveira, DDS
   Barbro Svensson
   Rehabilitaion Hospital of Bauru-USP
   Bauru-USP, Brazil

3 Richard Babin, MD
   University of Iowa
   Iowa City, Iowa

4 Gordon Wilkes, MD
   Compru-Misericordia Hospital
   Edmonton, Canada

5 Gordon Wilkes, MD
   Compru-Misericordia Hospital
   Edmonton, Canada

6 Michael Goldman, MD
   Leslie Heffez, DDS
   Henry O. Gold, DDS
   University of Illinois
   Chicago, Illinois

7 José Maria Diaz Torres, MD
   Madrid, Spain

8 Michael J. Wake, MD
   David Proops, MD
   Queen Elizabeth Hospital
   Birmingham, UK

Key to Clinicians

The clinical cases in Part I are presented using the anaplastologists initials as given:

(AF) Ann Fyler
(AR) Ann-Marie Riedinger-Keller
(DM) David C. Macnamara
(DT) David Trainer
(ED) Enrique de Damborenea
(GD) Gillian F. Duncan
(GG) Gregory G. Gion
(IH) Irene Healey
(IM) Iain Mathieson
(JB) Julie Jordan Brown
(JW) Johan Wolfaardt
(KB) Kerstin Bergström
(KT) Keith Thomas
(LM) Lou Ann Mercier
(PE) Peter Evans
(PS) Paula J. Sauerborn
(SG) Steven Gray
(SH) Susan Habakuk
(SW) Steve Worrollo

Patient Presentations

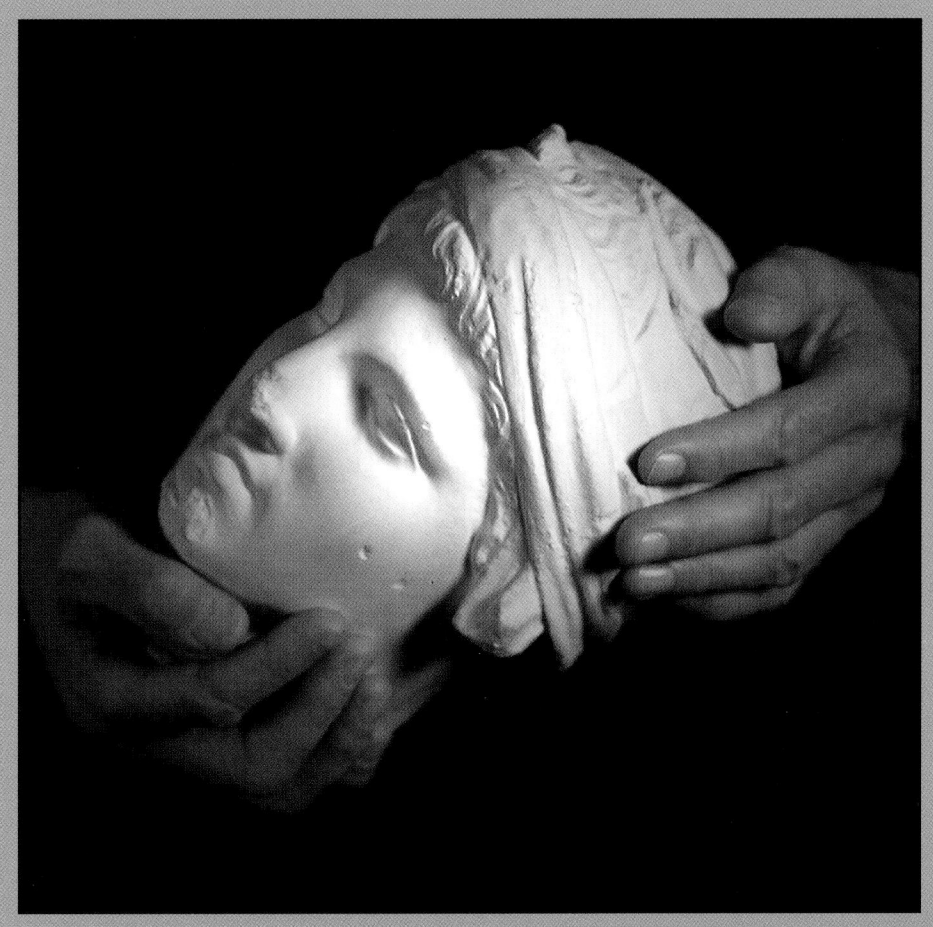

AURICULAR DEFECTS

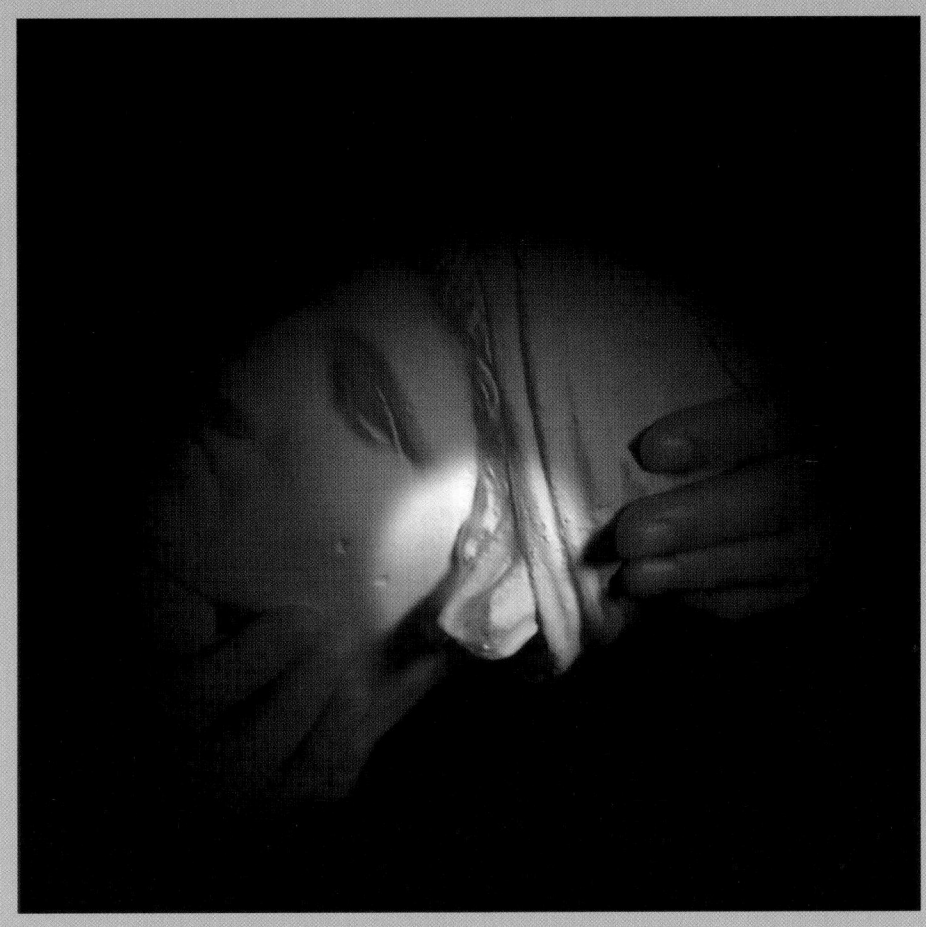

PATIENT PRESENTATION 1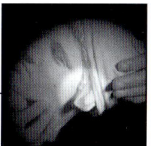

1 *This 8-year-old girl had bilateral atresia of the ears. Autogenous plastic surgical reconstruction was considered, but the family opted for prosthetic auricular reconstruction. Two fixtures were placed on each side to provide mechanical retention for the prosthesis, and a third fixture was placed on the right side for a bone-anchored hearing aid. About 3 weeks after the abutment connection, performed at a later stage, a gold bar was constructed onto the abutments, and the silicone auricular prosthesis was retained with clips incorporated into the acrylic plate. (KB)*

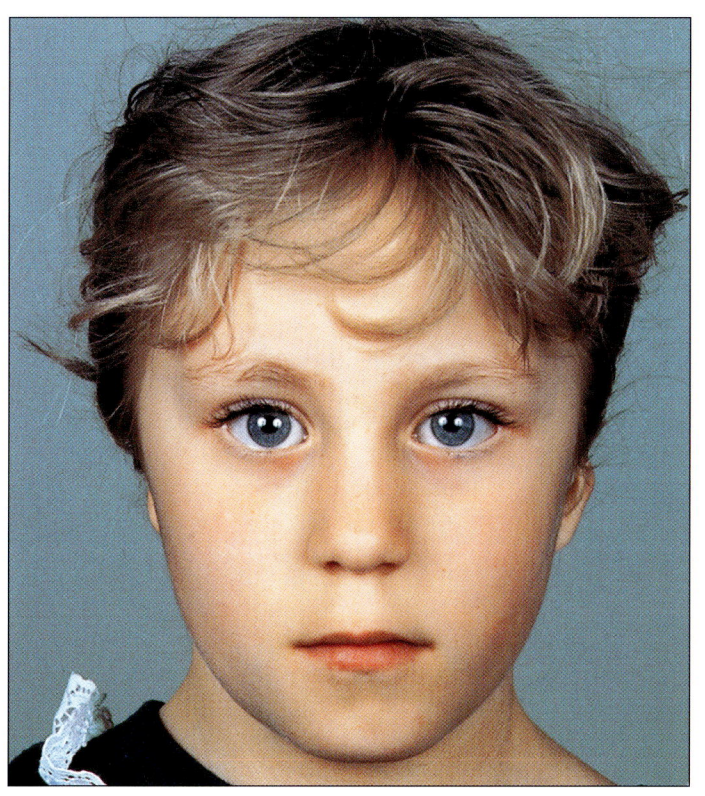
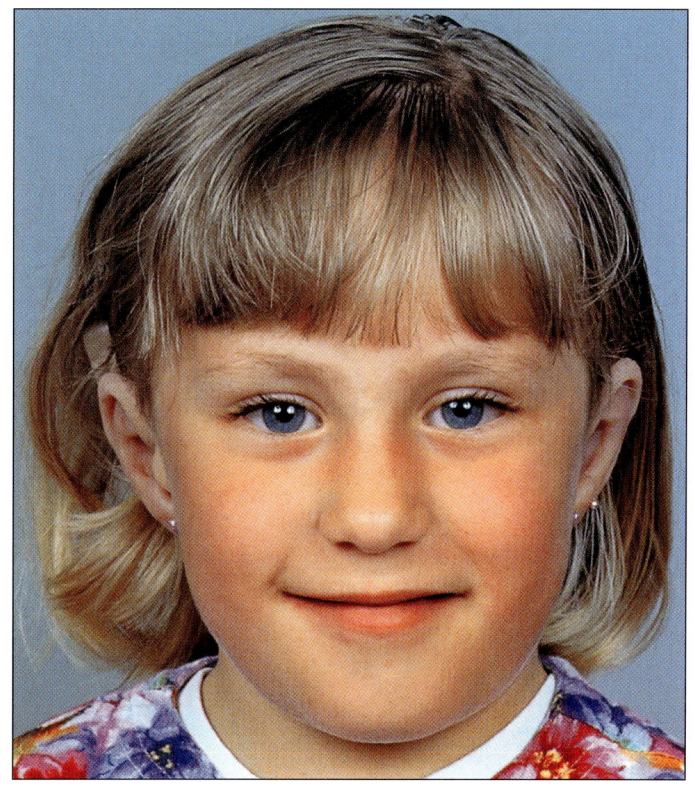
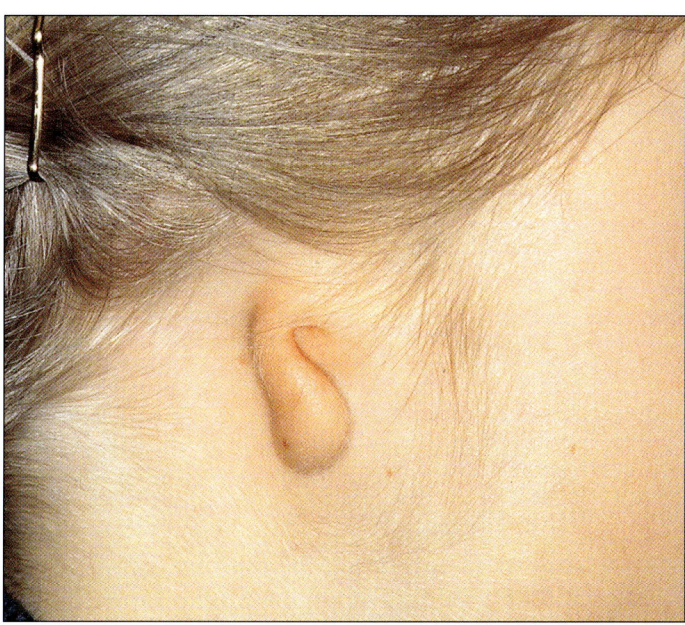
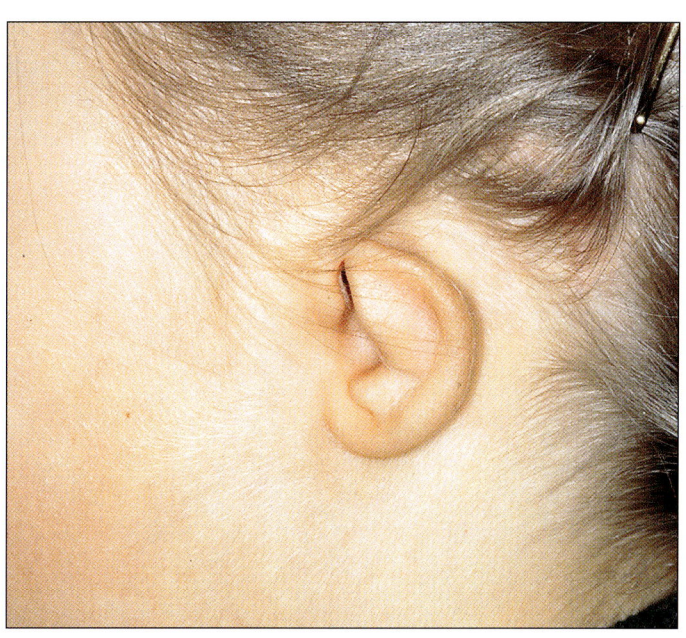

(continued)

Patient Presentation 1

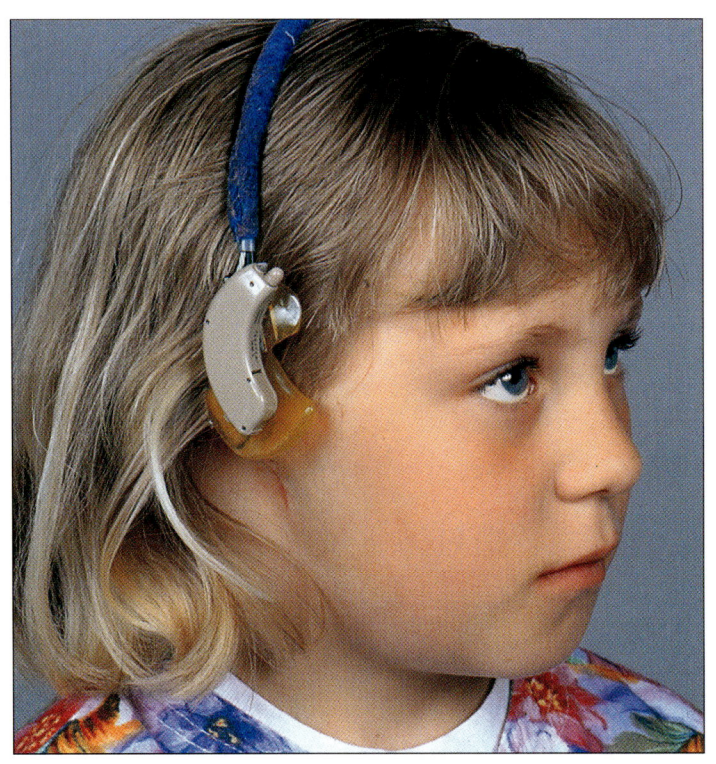
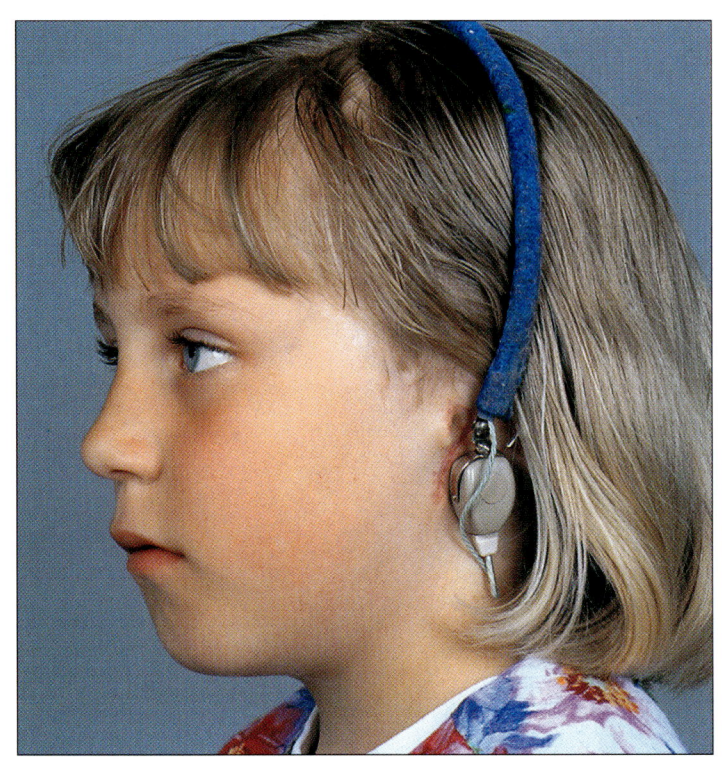
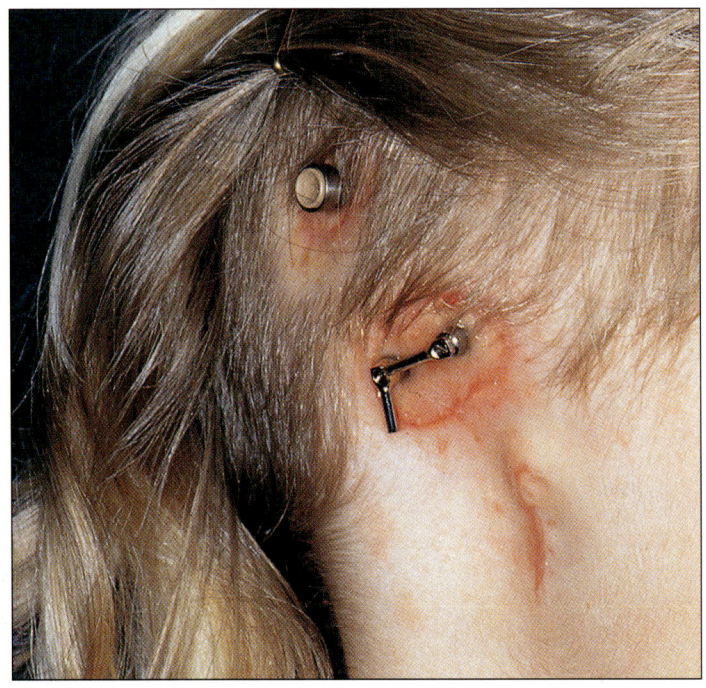
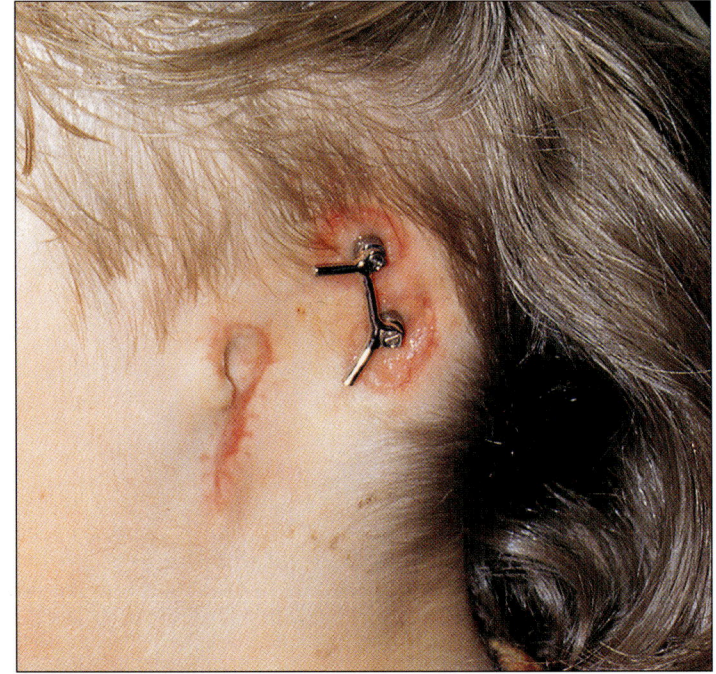

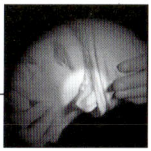

PATIENT PRESENTATION 1

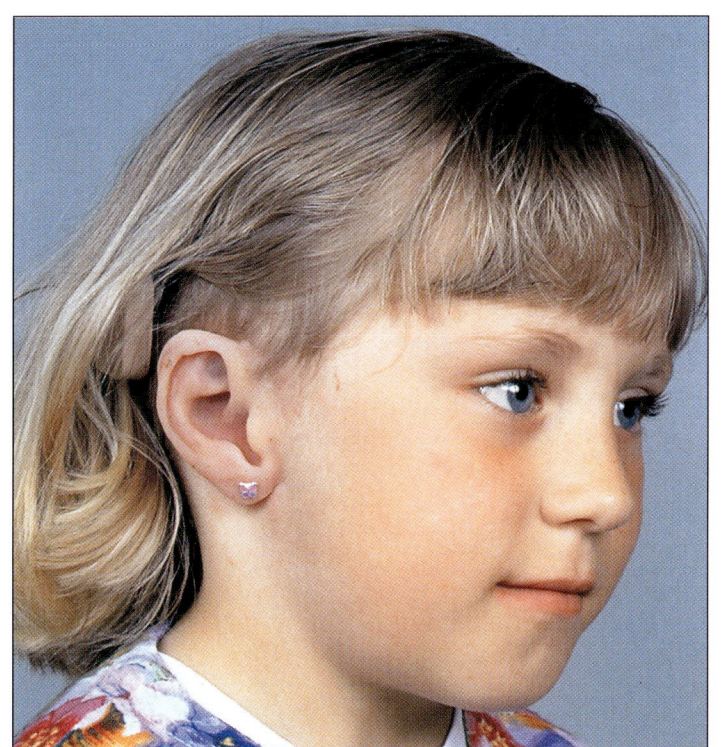
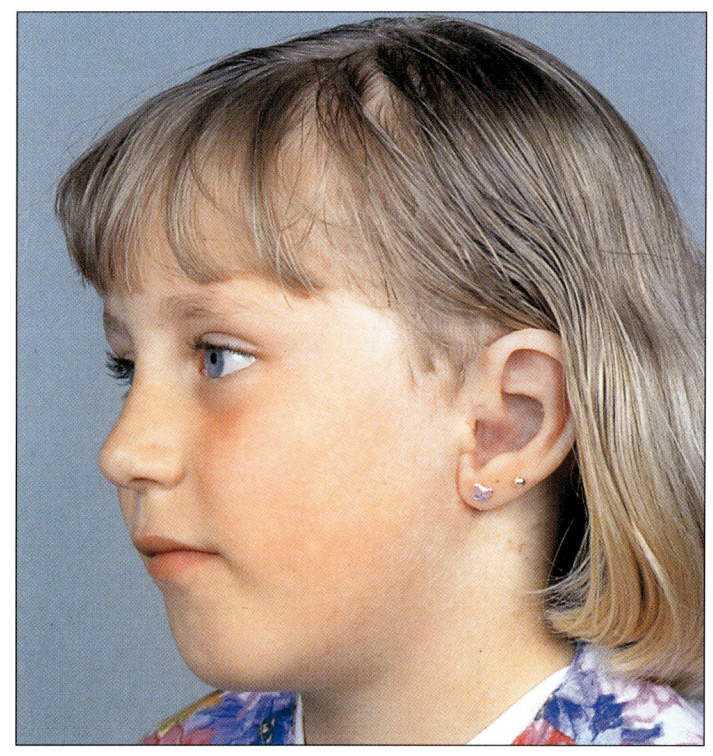
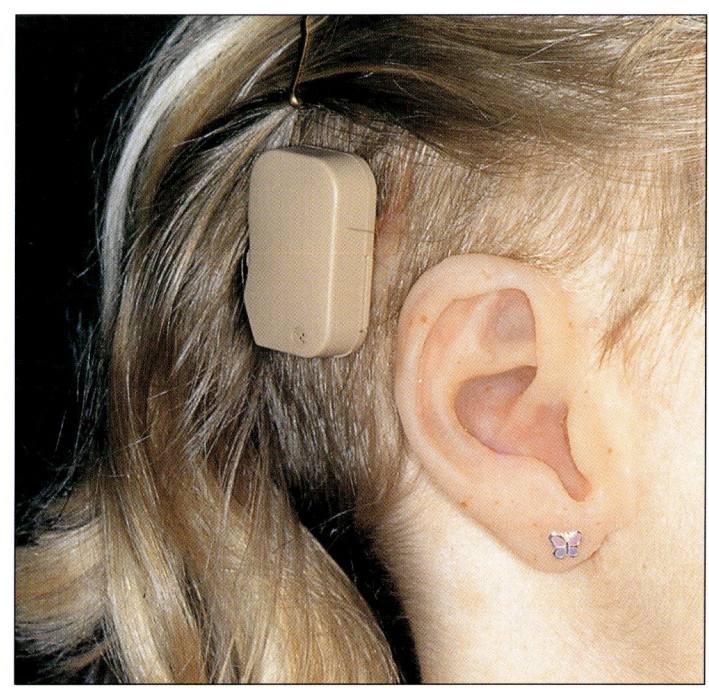

PATIENT PRESENTATION 2

2 *This 54-year-old man suffered a traumatic amputation of the right ear. A silicone auricular prosthesis was fabricated, restoring the missing facial structure. (JB)*

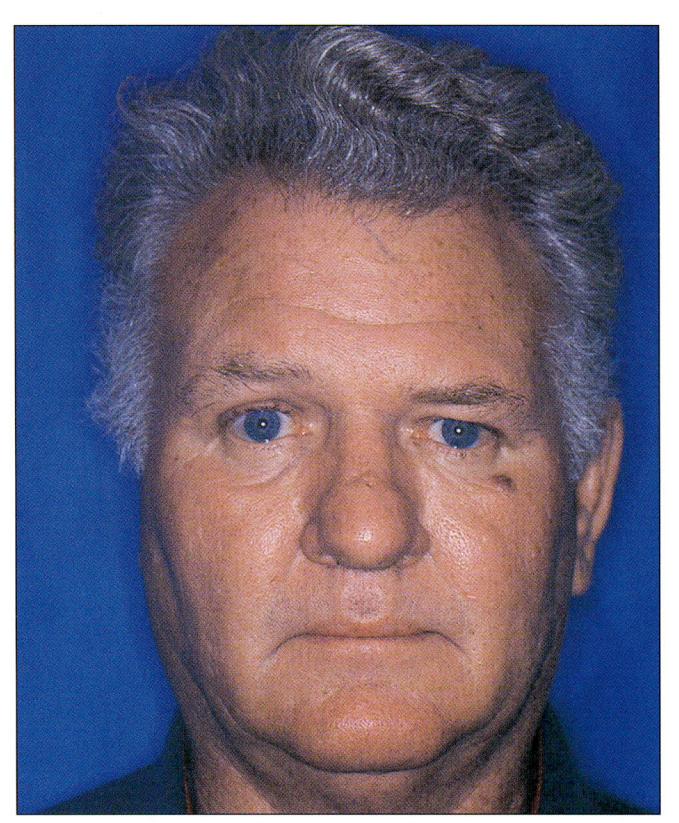
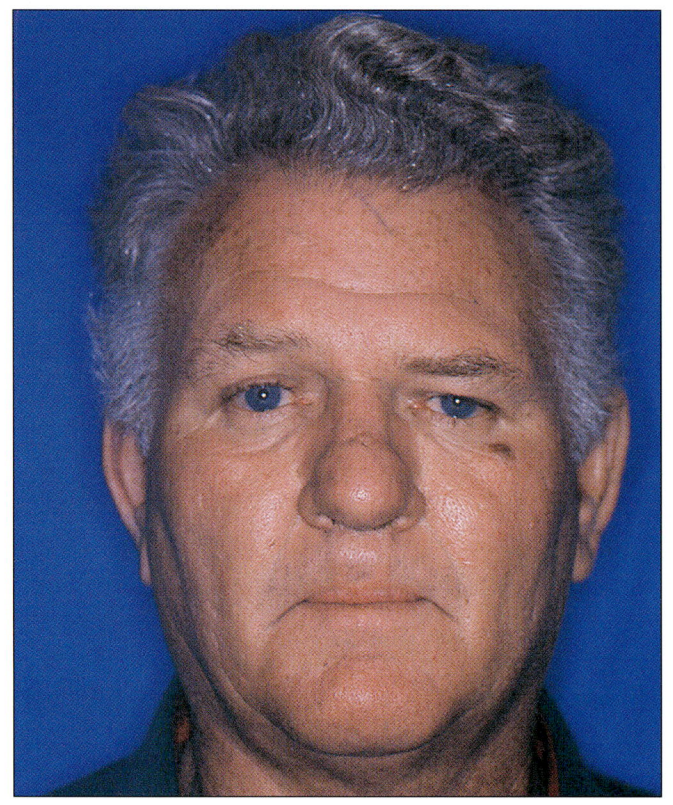
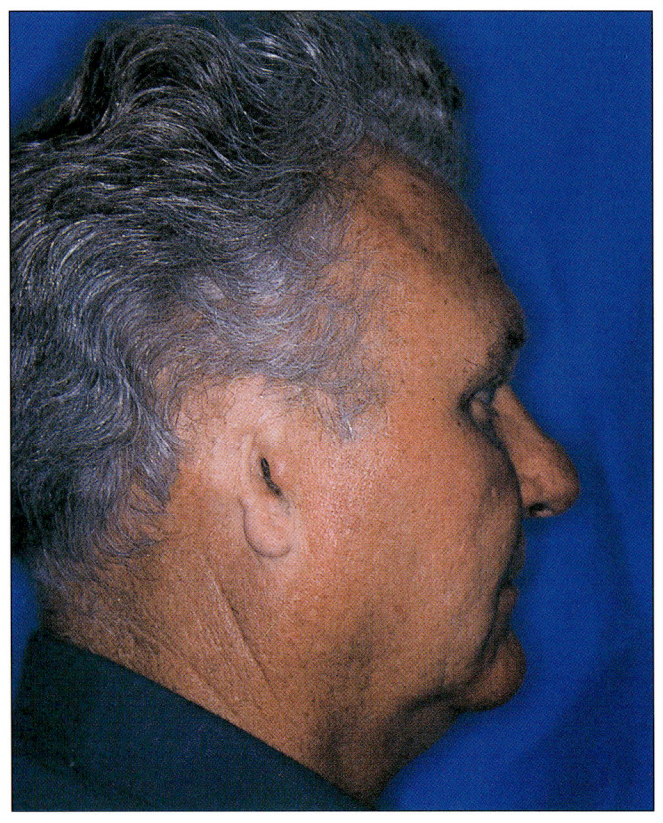
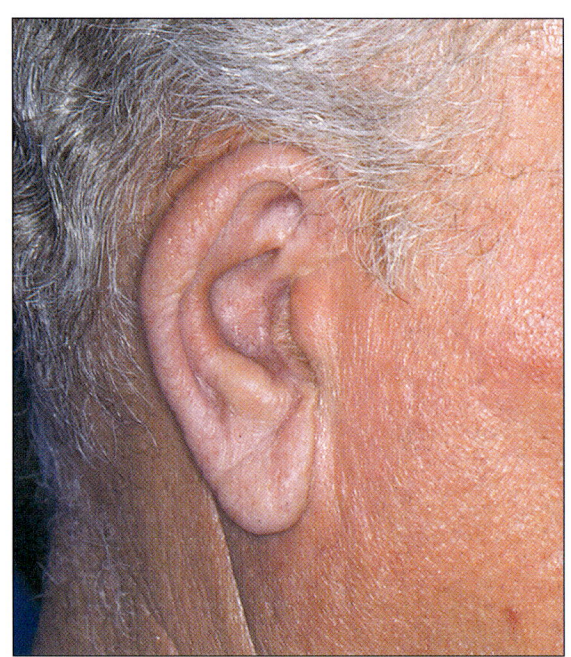

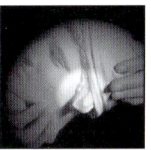

3 *These figures show selected prosthetic steps for rehabilitation of a left auriculectomy due to squamous cell carcinoma. Initially, the prosthesis was anchored on two fixtures, but the final results were not satisfactory because of a gap on the front edge. To provide a larger base plate, three more fixtures were placed. Magnets were used instead of a bar for easier cleaning of the prosthesis. The base plate was split and sprung to keep the front edge in contact with the skin and to reduce stress on the implants. (PE)*

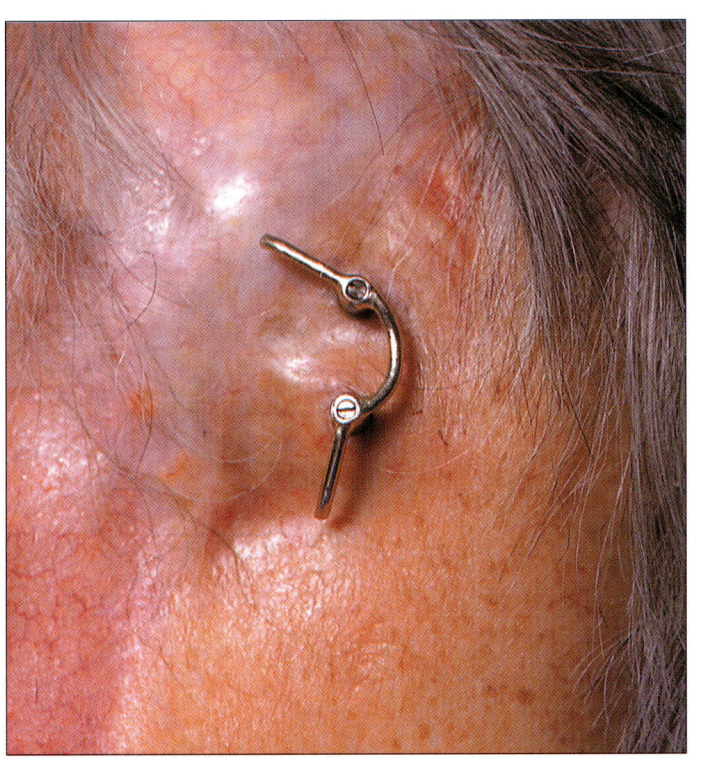
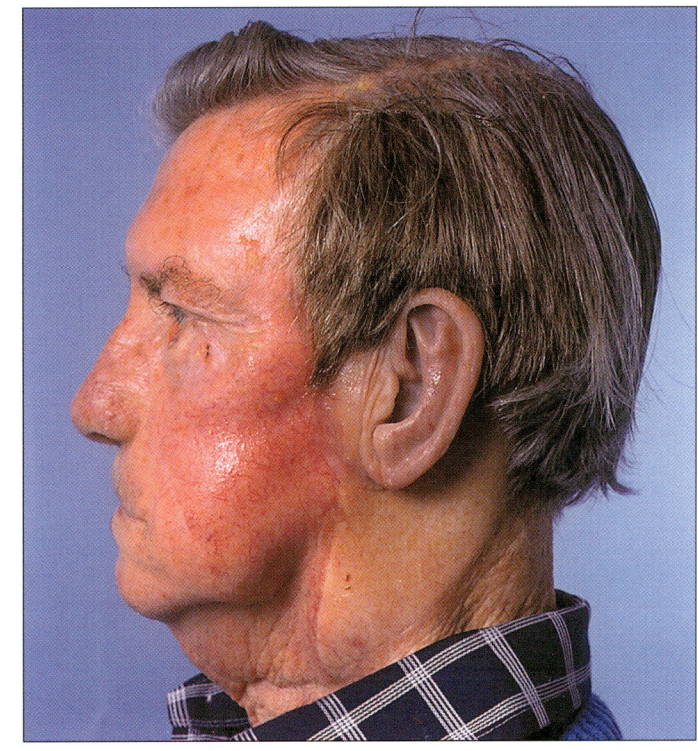
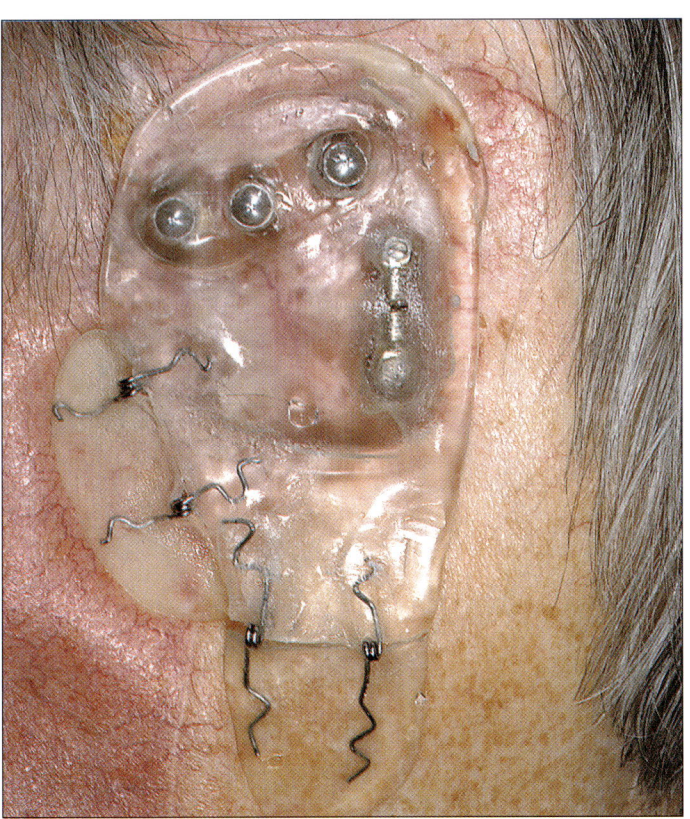
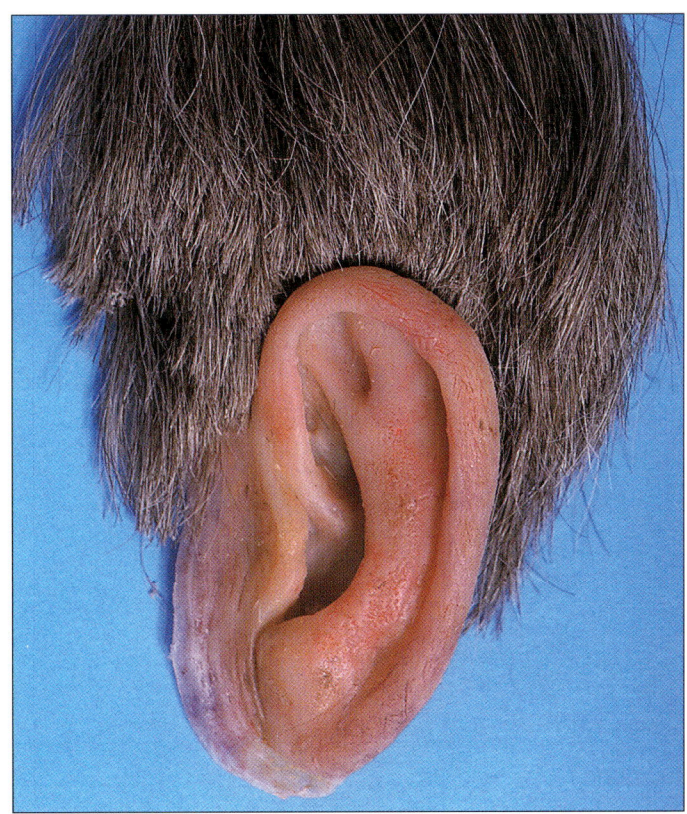

Patient Presentation 4

4 *This 58-year-old man underwent a traumatic amputation of the right ear in a car accident. He was provided with an adhesive-retained silicone prosthesis. (AF)*

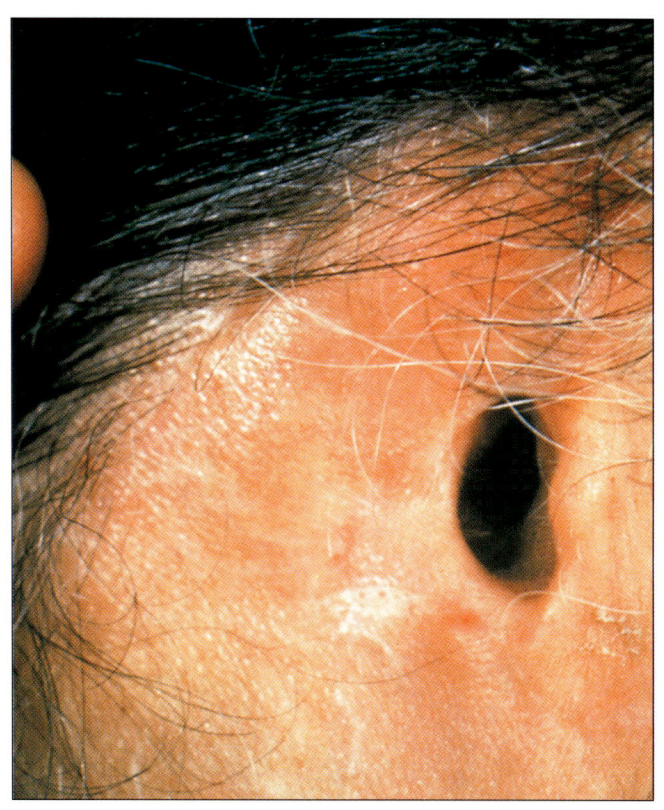
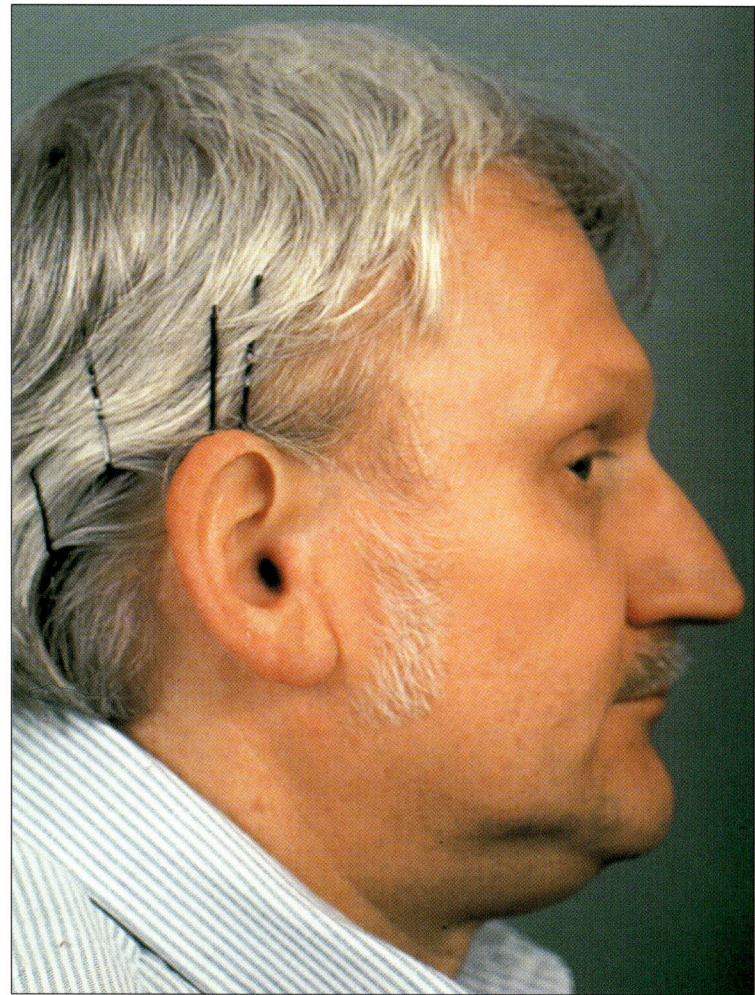

PATIENT PRESENTATION 5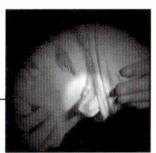

5 This 61-year-old man underwent a right auriculectomy due to squamous cell carcinoma. After the healing period, an adhesive-retained silicone auricular prosthesis was provided. (GG)

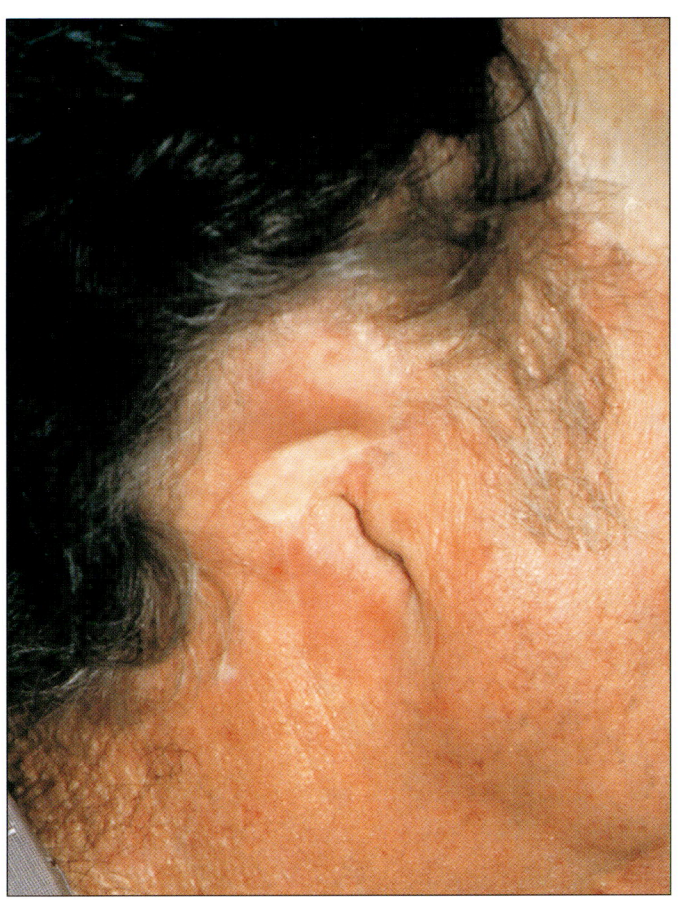
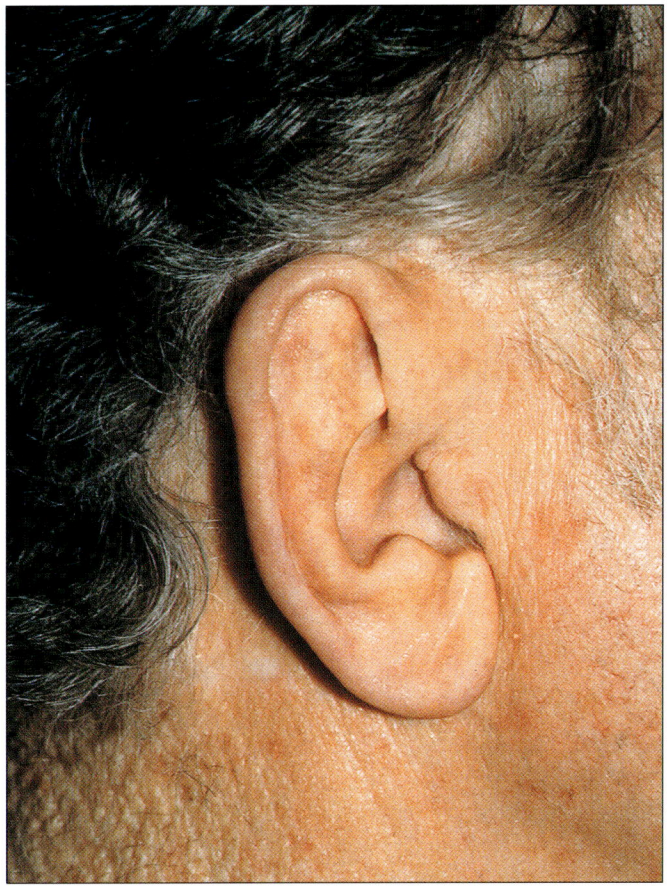
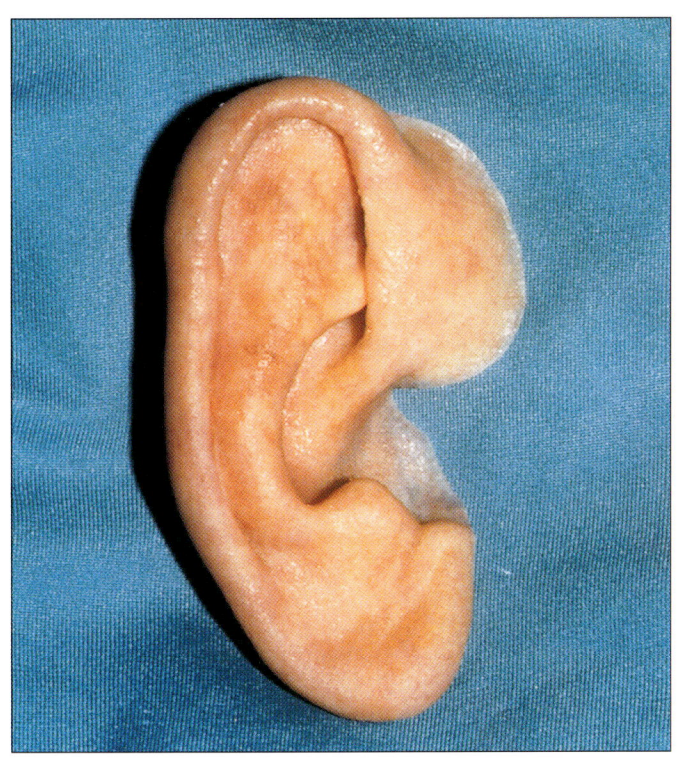

PATIENT PRESENTATION 6

6 *This 62-year-old man suffered severe burns, which led to the loss of his right ear in 1963. He wore an artificial prosthesis for several years, and many problems due to skin sensitivity to the adhesive occurred. When he learned about the possibility of a bone-anchored prosthesis, he did not hesitate to submit to this treatment. The surgical procedures were performed in November 1992 (first stage), and in the beginning of 1993 for the second stage. After the healing period, a silicone auricular prosthesis with gold clips was retained to the gold bar fabricated onto the abutments. Since then, the patient has had no problems related to allergies or retention. (AR)*

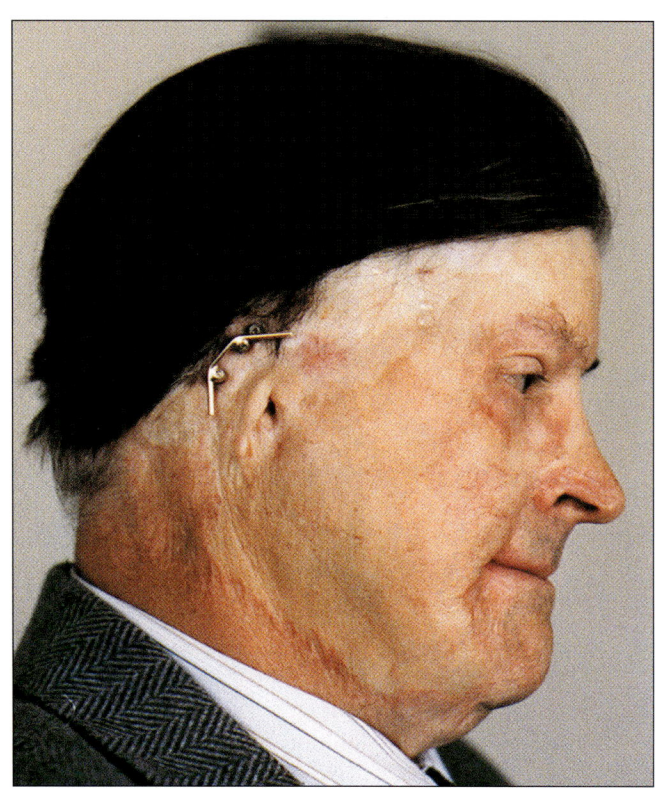
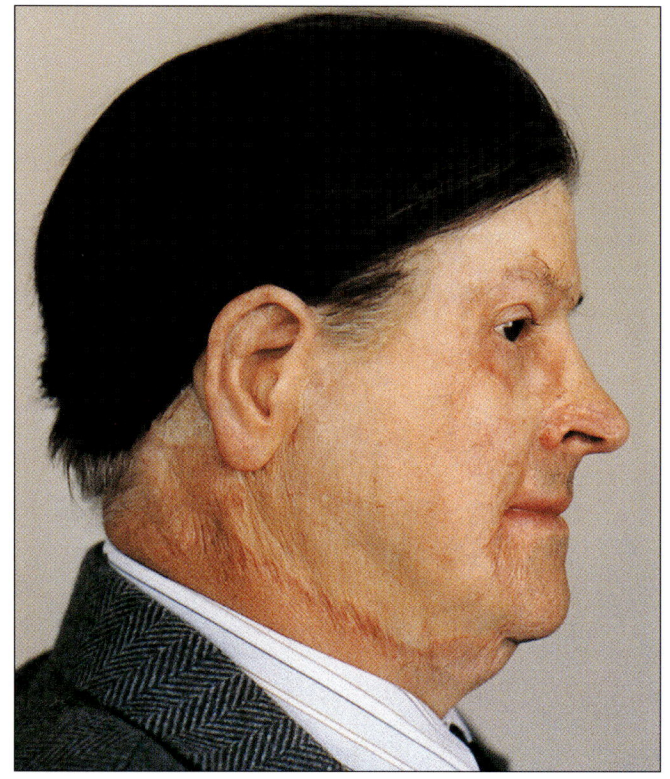
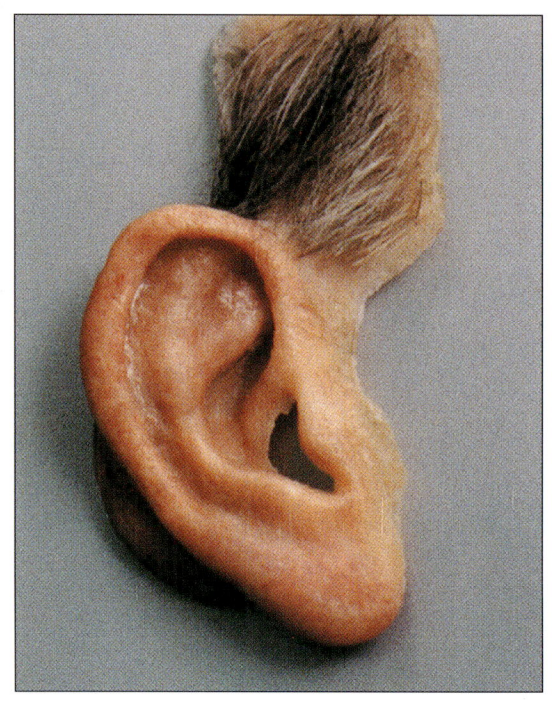

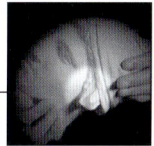

7 This 32-year-old man suffered a traumatic amputation of his left ear in a mining accident. Plastic surgery for reconstruction of the damaged ear was performed, but the result was not acceptable to the patient, who decided to wear a silicone prosthesis over the reconstructed ear. After several years, he opted for a bone-anchored prosthesis. Two fixtures were placed in the mastoid area, and abutments were connected at second-stage surgery. When the soft tissue had healed, a silicone auricular prosthesis was fabricated and retained to the gold bar with clips. (AR)

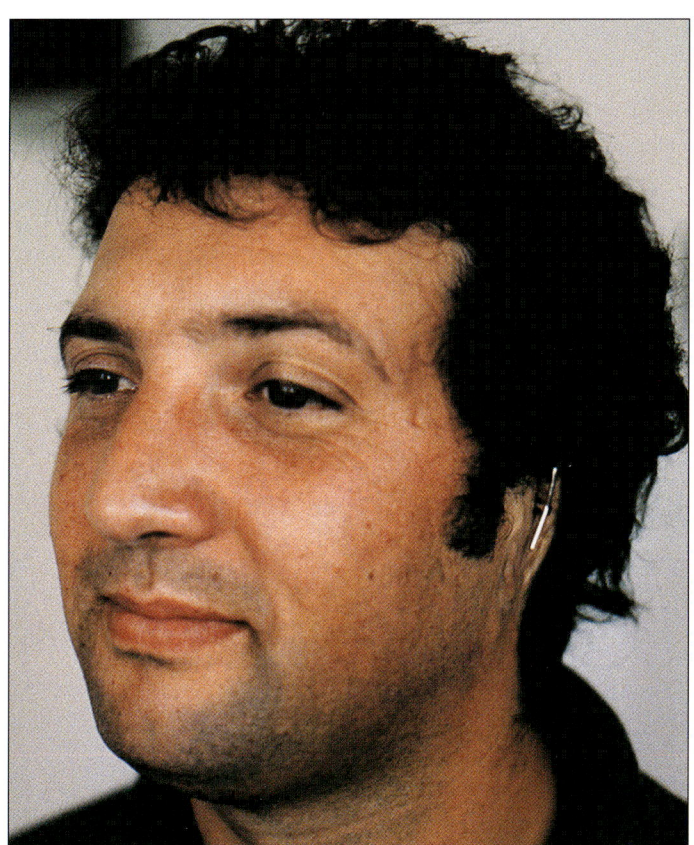
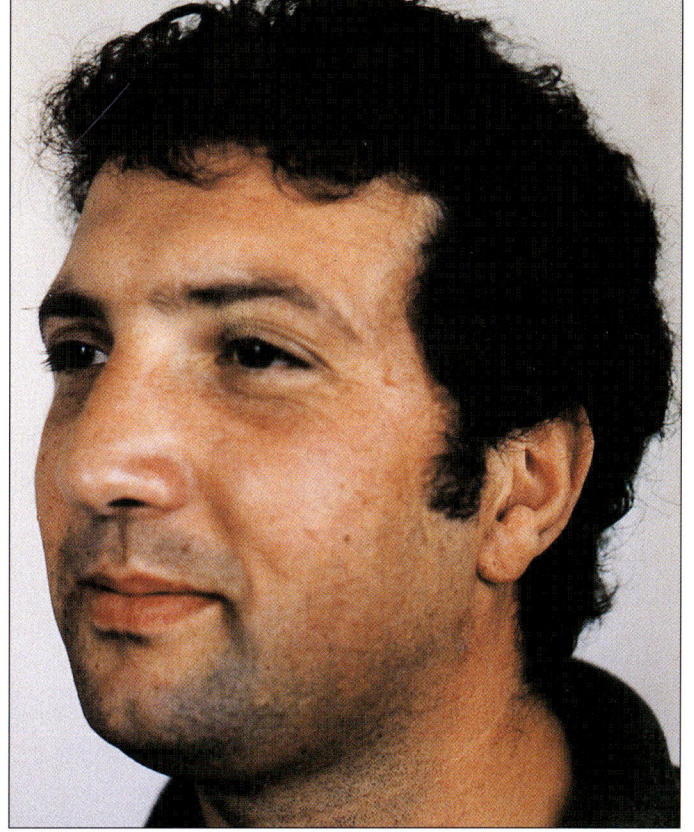
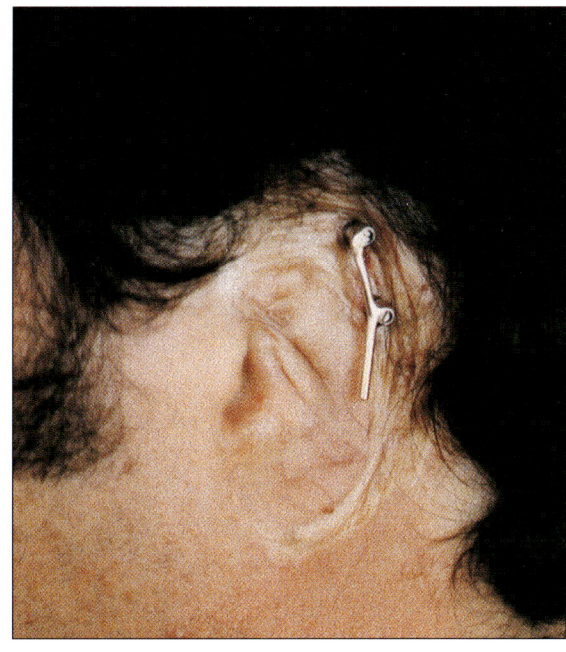

PATIENT PRESENTATION 8

8 *This 10-year-old girl was born with right hemifacial microsomia. The external auditory meatus was located 22 mm anterior and 17 mm inferior to the normal contralateral ear. When she was 5 years old, two fixtures were placed to provide mechanical retention for the prosthesis. After the abutment connection, performed at a later stage, a gold bar was fabricated onto the abutments, and the silicone auricular prosthesis was retained with gold clips. (PS)*

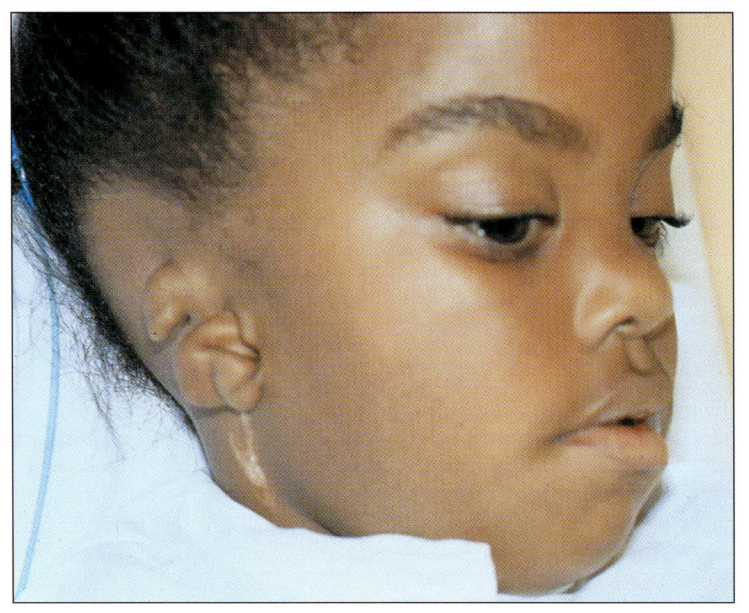
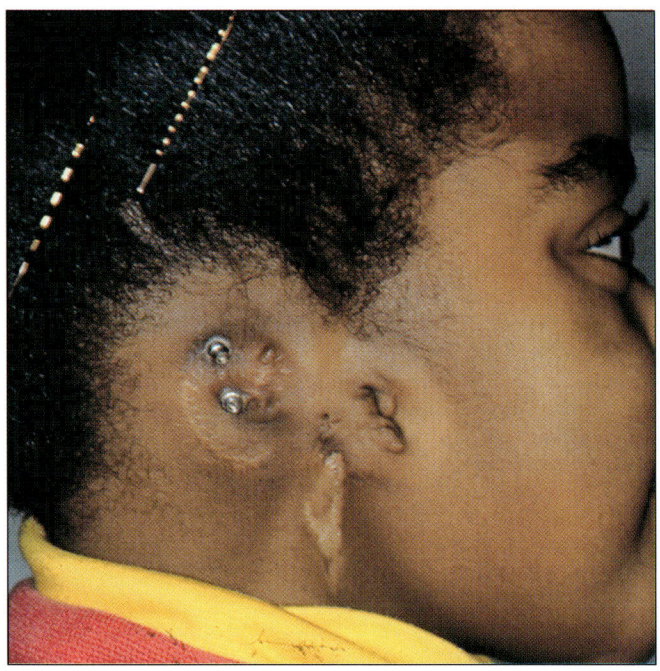
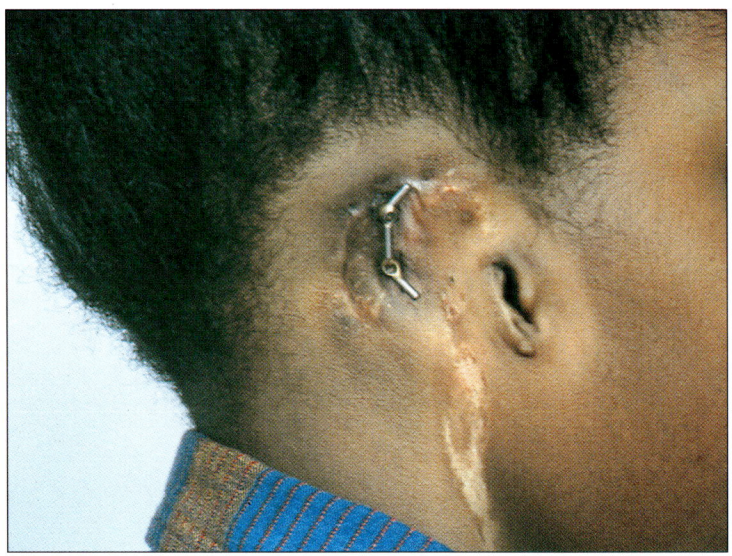
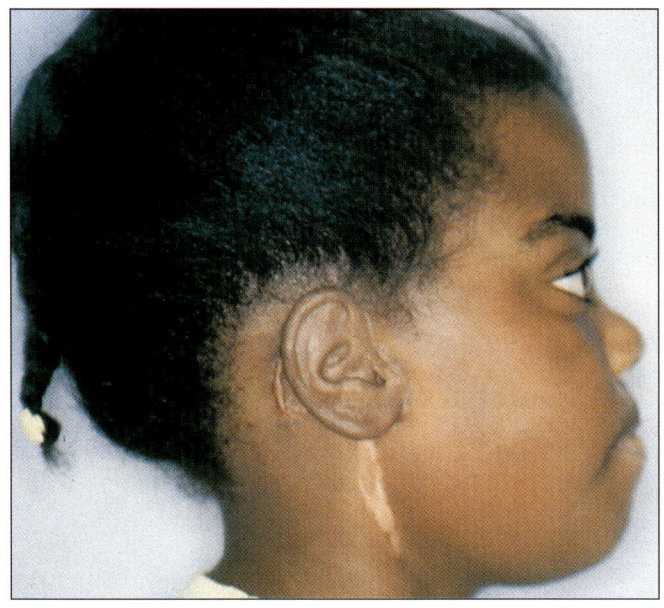

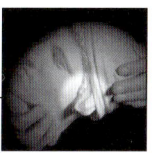

9 This 66-year-old man underwent a total pinnectomy due to a large fungating lesion of the right pinna. He opted for a bone-anchored auricular prosthesis, so two fixtures were placed in the mastoid area. Since this procedure was performed in one stage, two 4-mm abutments were connected to the fixtures. Three months later, an impression of the area was made, and a 2-mm round gold bar was constructed and soldered to the 4-mm gold cylinders. The silicone auricular prosthesis was retained to the bar by three gold clips incorporated into the acrylic plate of the prosthesis. (KT)

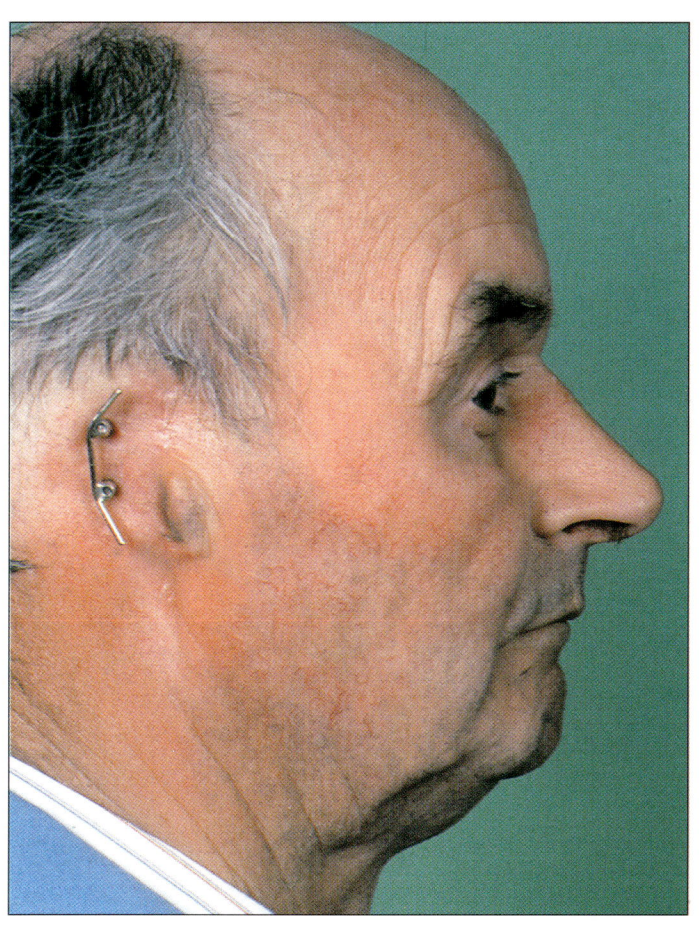
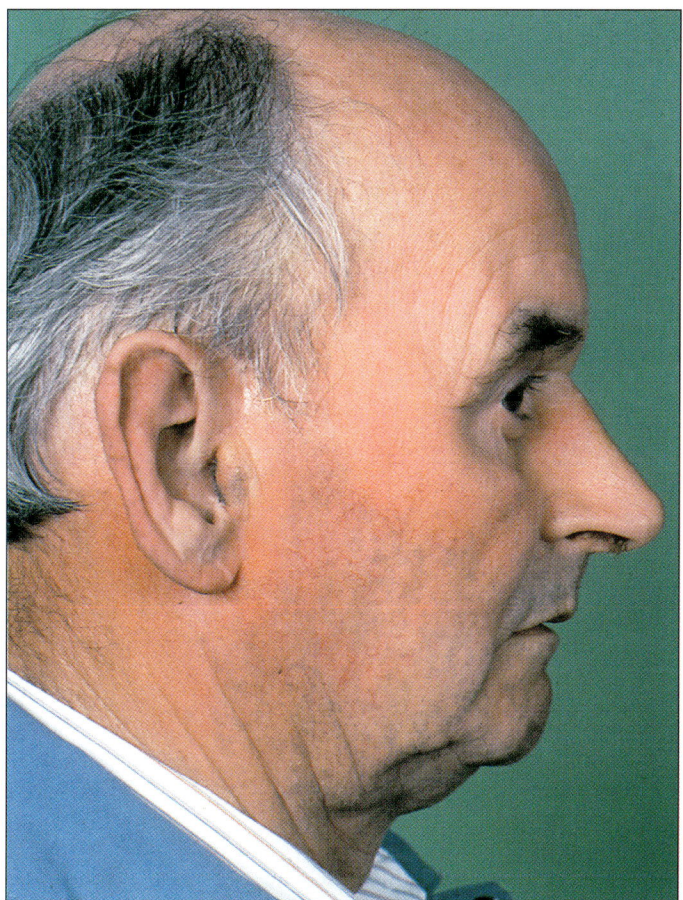

PATIENT PRESENTATION 10

10 *This 20-year-old man was born with a right auricular deformity. Two fixtures were placed in the mastoid area, providing mechanical retention for the silicone auricular prosthesis. (DT)*

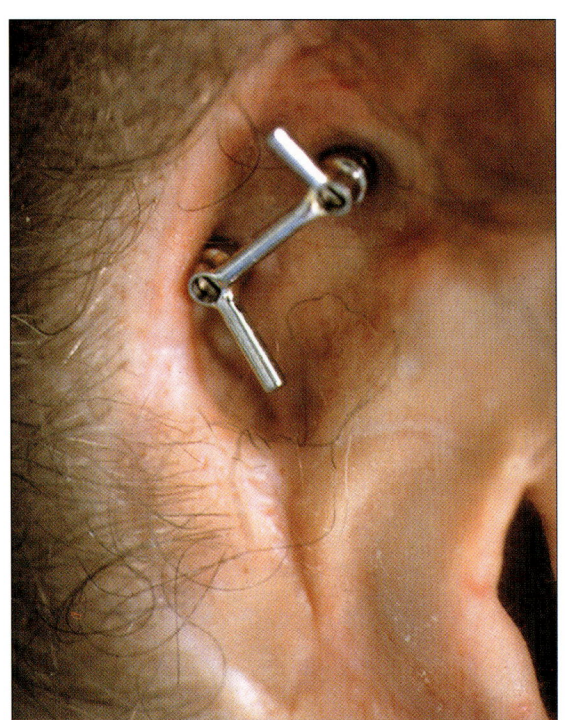
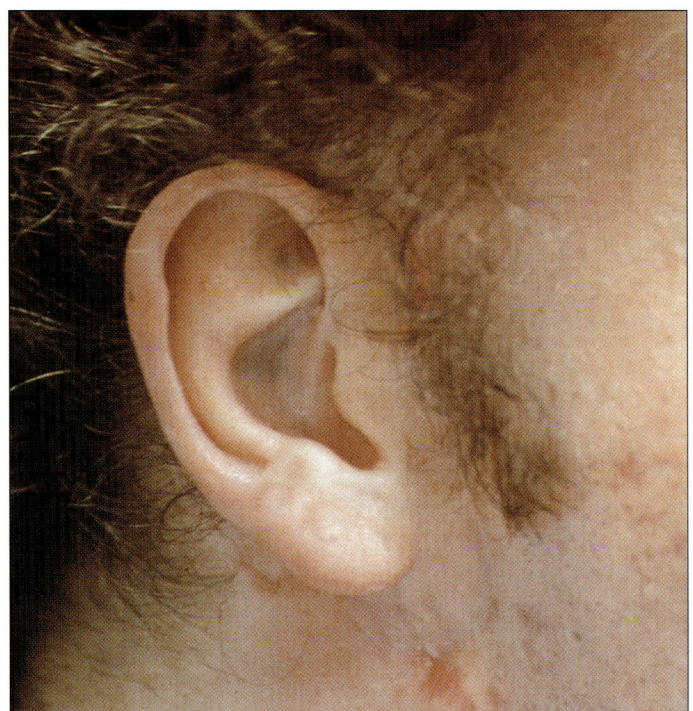
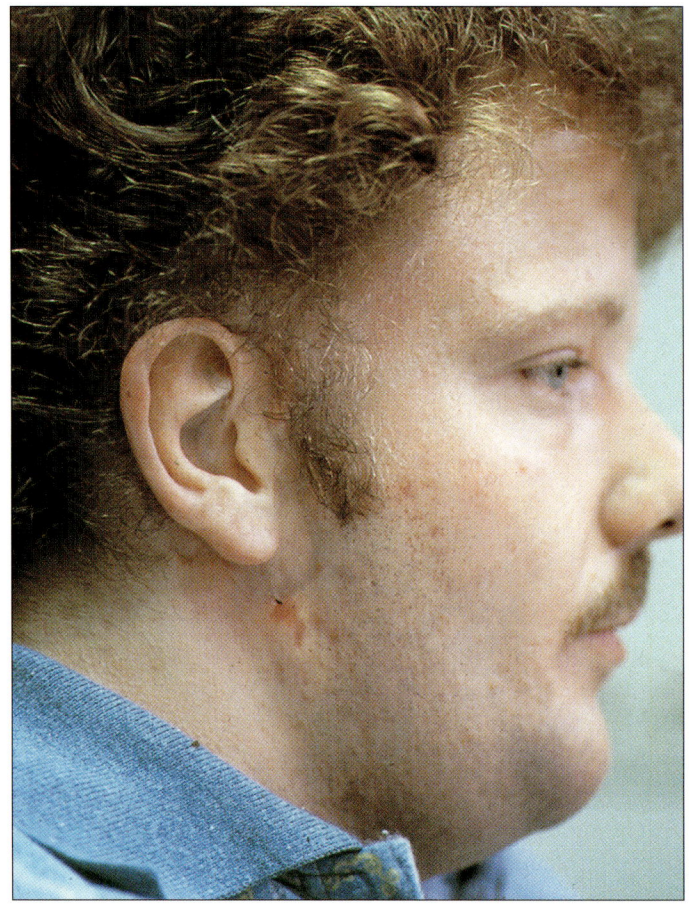

PATIENT PRESENTATION 11

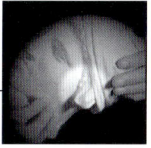

11 *This young woman underwent multiple procedures for right auricular reconstruction of a microtia. The patient history indicated that a silicone elastomer framework had been used in the reconstruction of the auricle. The result was unacceptable to the patient, who elected to undergo reconstruction with a bone-anchored auricular prosthesis. The silicone elastomer framework was removed, and the tissue bed in the area of the prosthesis was recontoured. Two fixtures were placed to retain the prosthesis on a bar-and-clip system. (JW)*

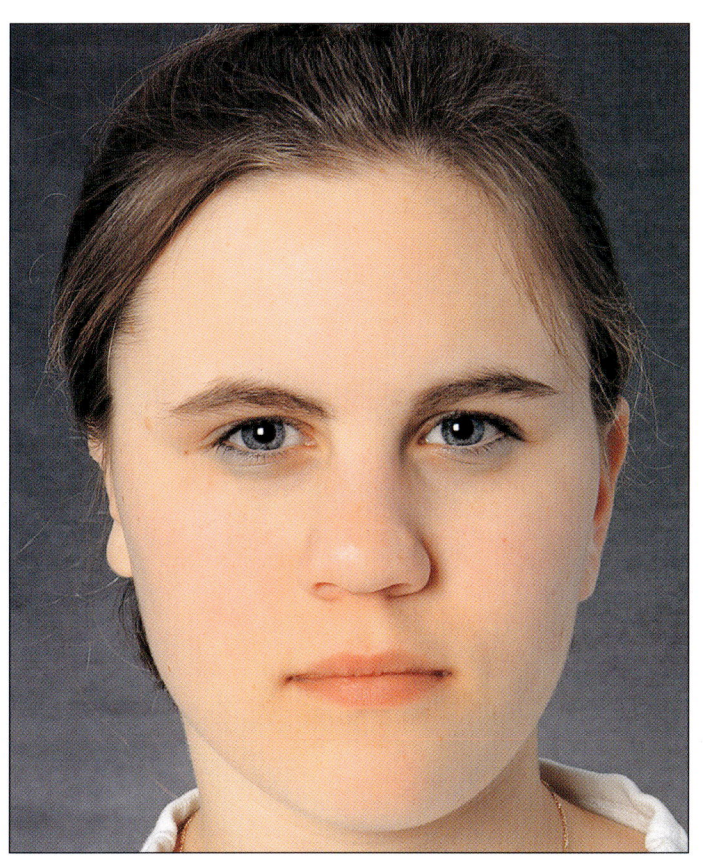
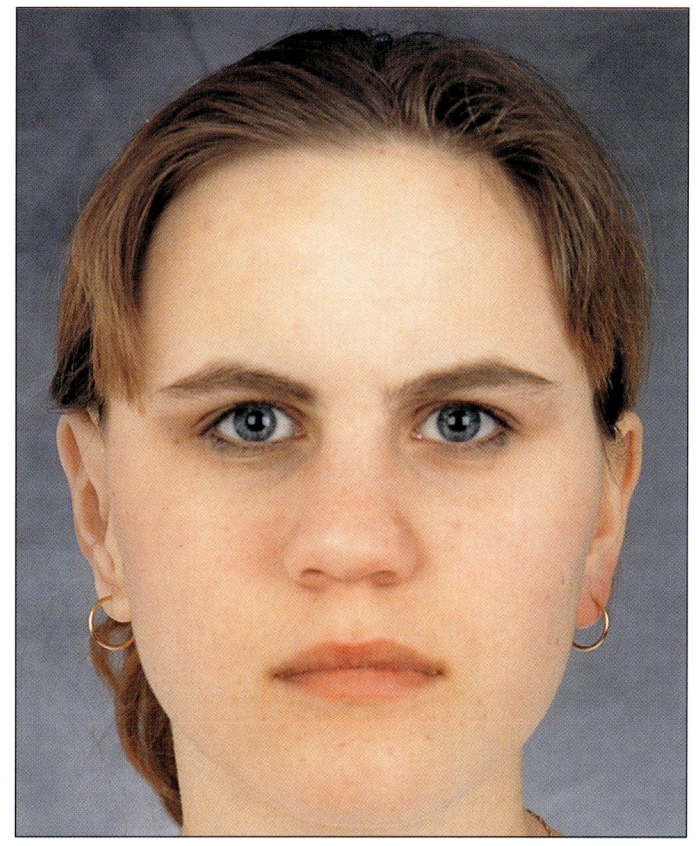
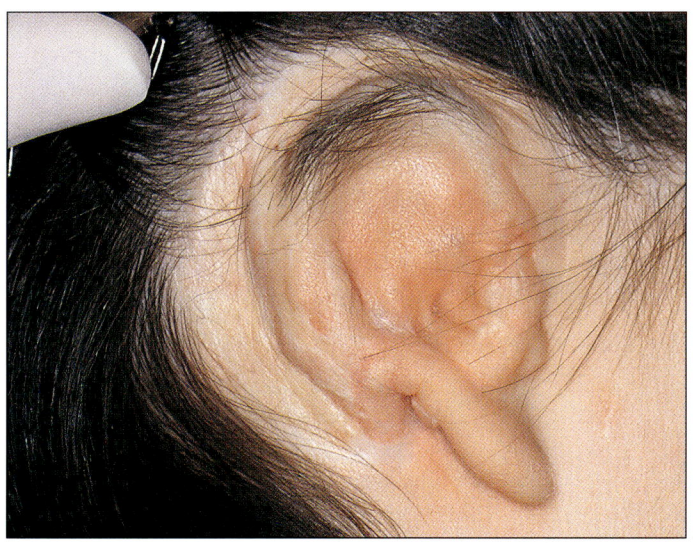
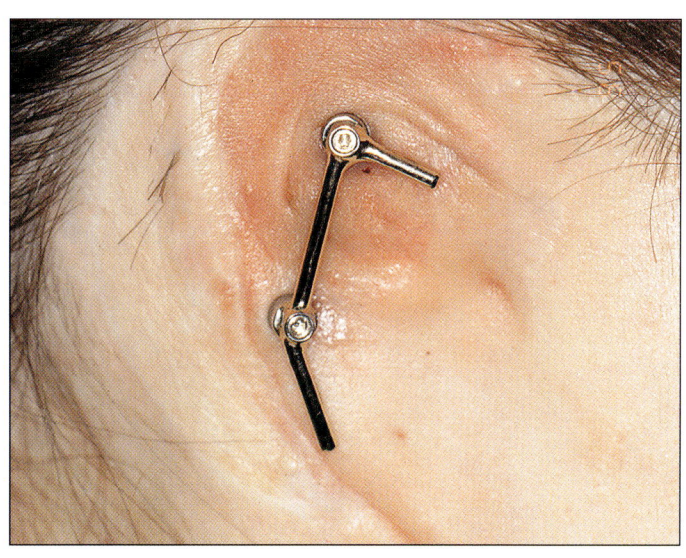

(continued)

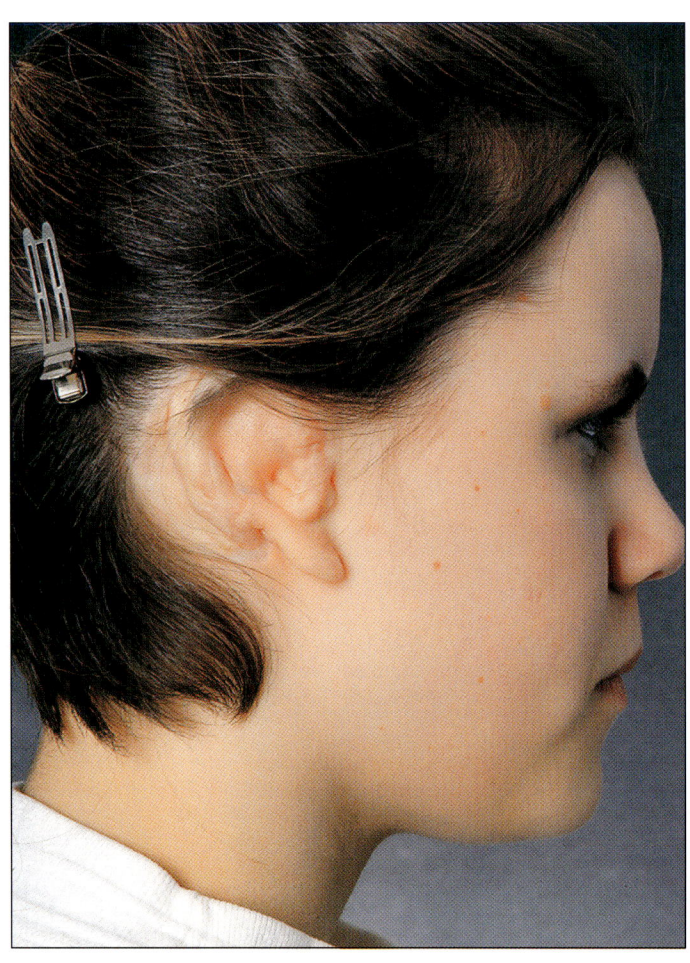
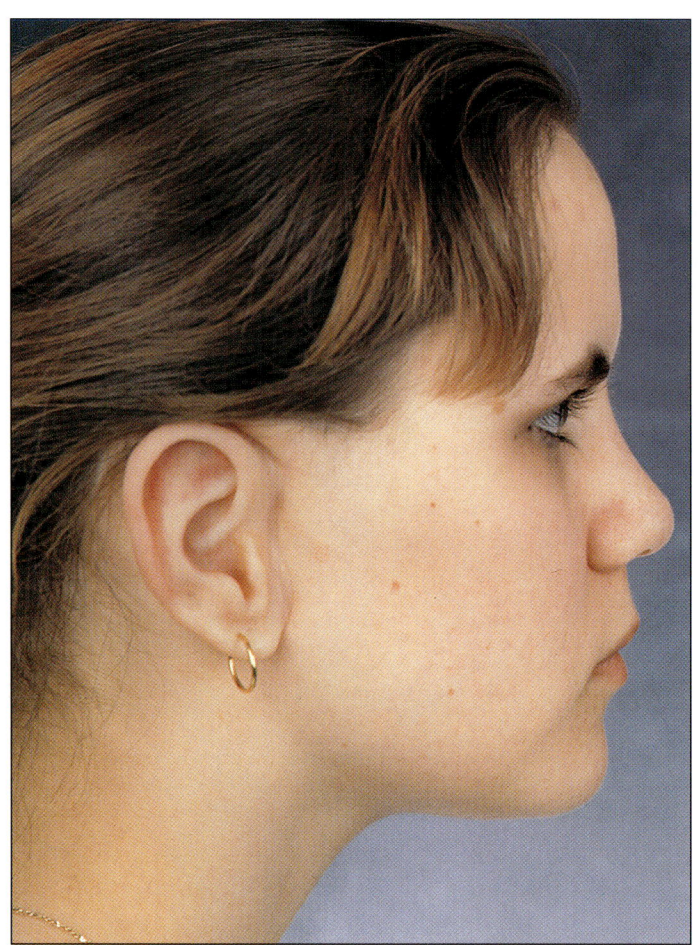
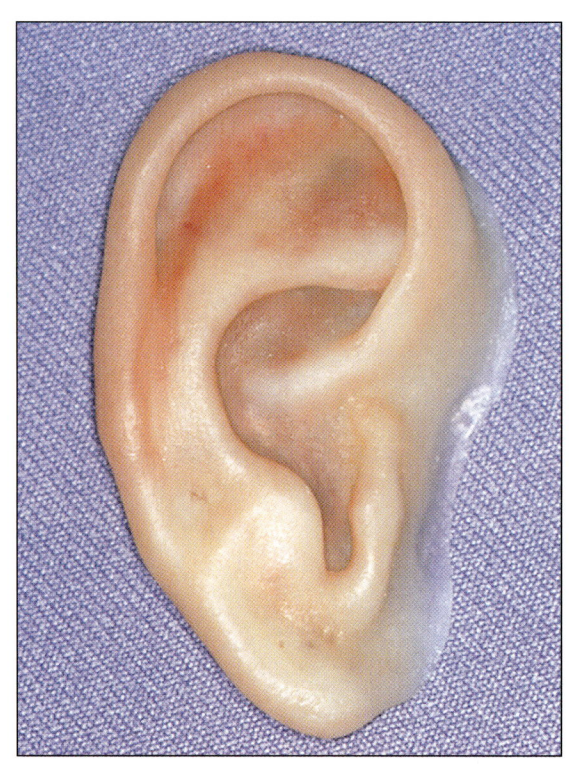

PATIENT PRESENTATION 12

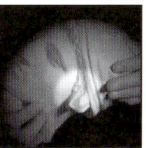

12 This 70-year-old man underwent a right auriculectomy due to a large fungating lesion on the pinna. Since he decided to have a bone-anchored prosthesis, two fixtures were placed in the mastoid area immediately after the resection of the ear. At a second-stage procedure, abutments were connected to the fixtures, and 2 months later a clip-retained silicone auricular prosthesis was fitted, restoring the missing facial structure. (SW)

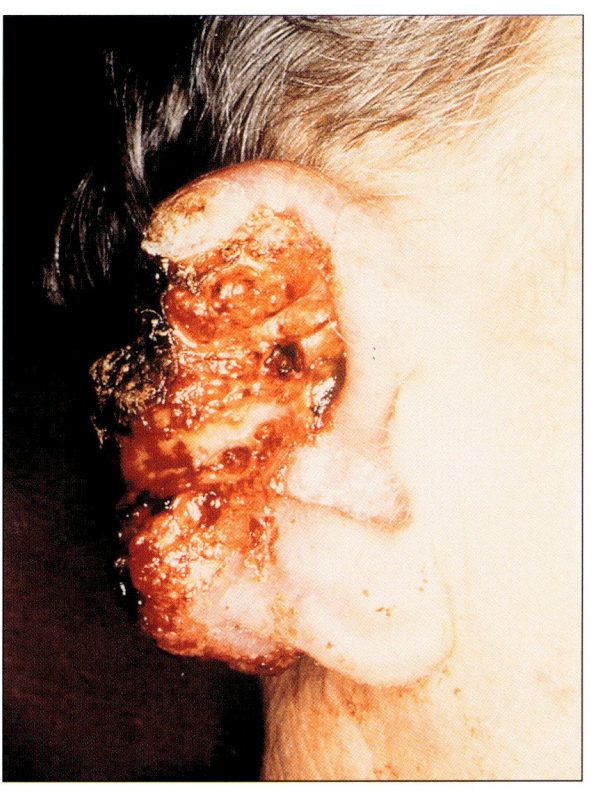

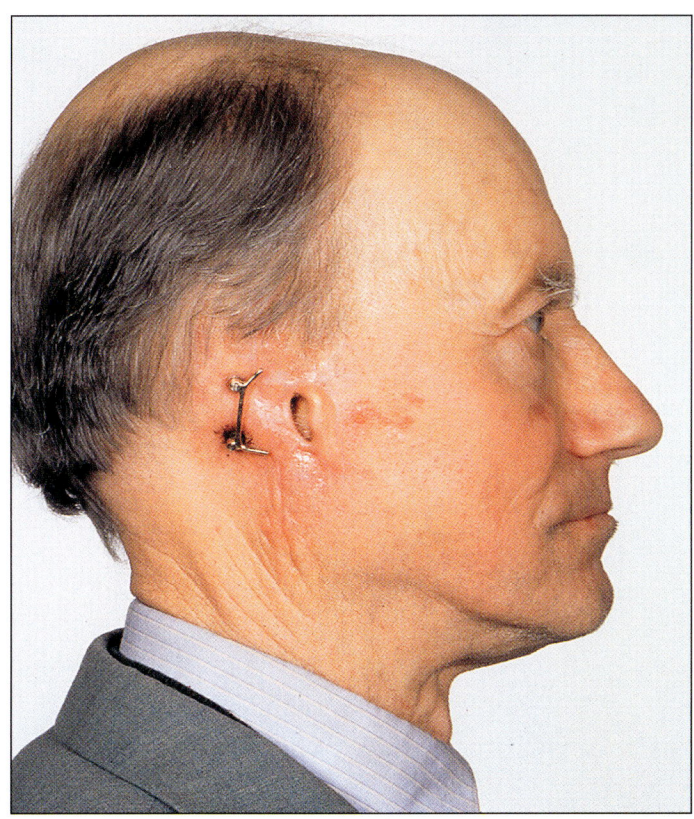

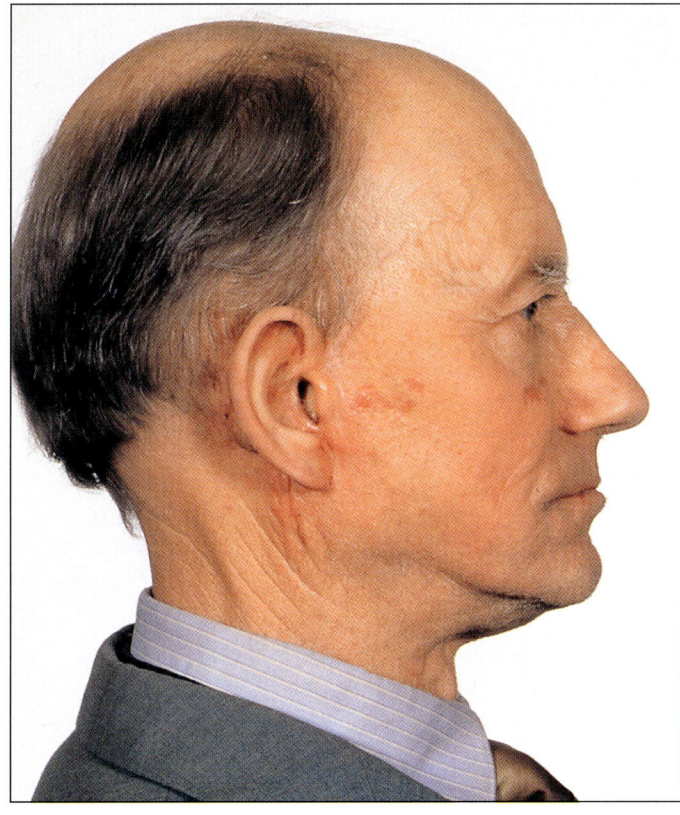

13 *This 23-year-old man suffered traumatic amputation of his right ear in a motor vehicle accident. He decided to have a bone-anchored auricular prosthesis, so three 4.0-mm fixtures were placed in the mastoid area. After the healing period, two of the fixtures were exposed by 5.5-mm abutments. A gold bar was constructed, and the silicone auricular prosthesis was retained by clips. In this case, the prosthesis was fabricated from medical adhesive 891. (IH)*

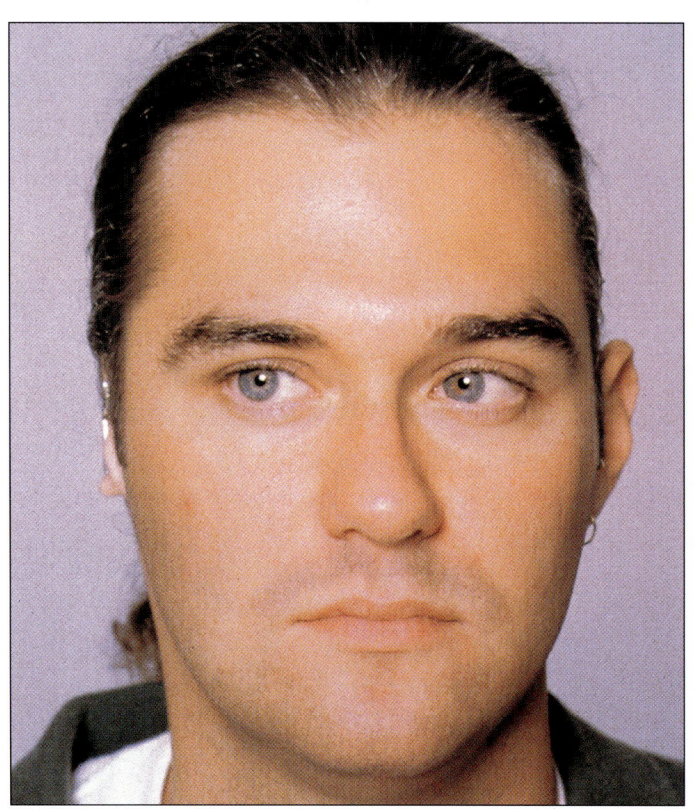
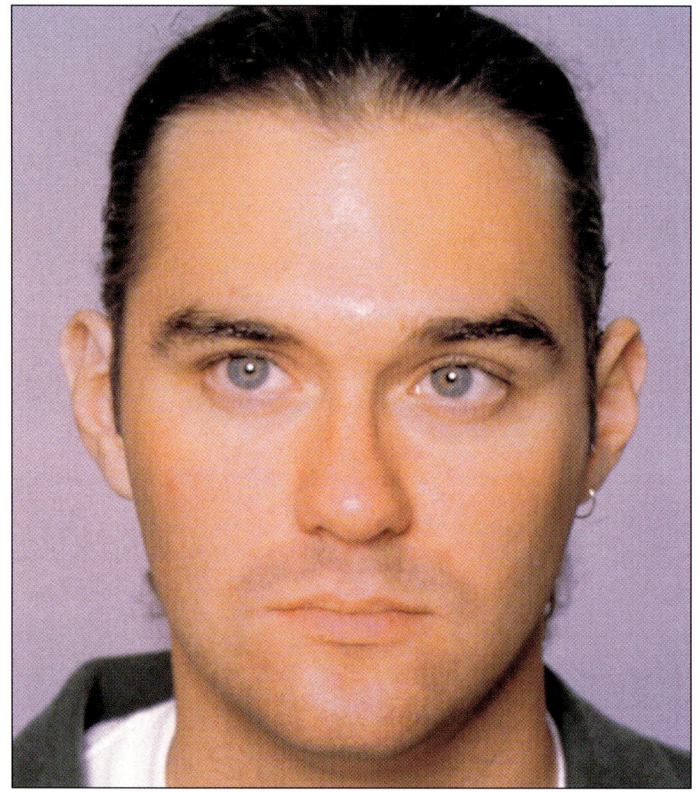
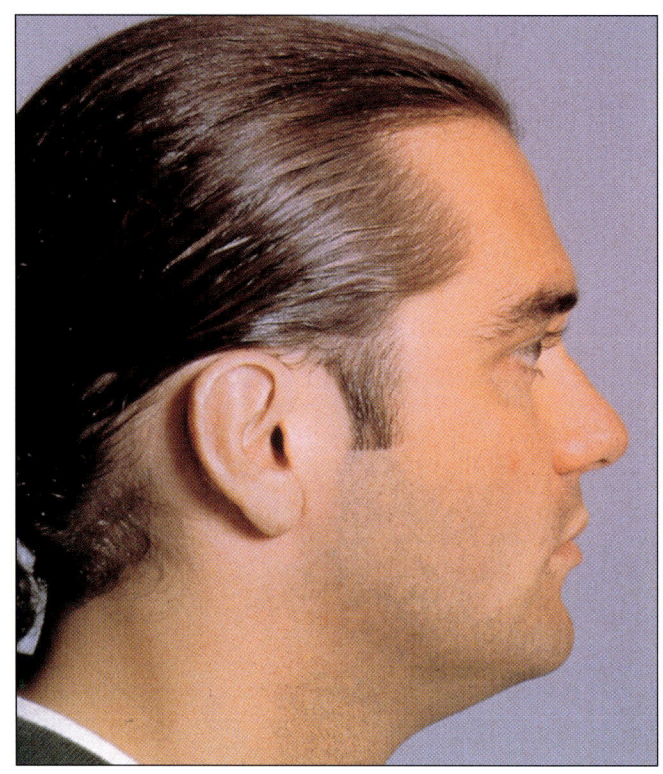

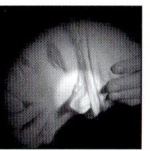

Patient Presentation 14

14 This 63-year-old man underwent a right auriculectomy due to a malignant melanoma in 1981. He was provided an adhesive-retained auricular prosthesis that was not acceptable to him. In 1990, a two-stage procedure was performed, and two fixtures were placed in the mastoid area to retain a bone-anchored auricular prosthesis with a bar-and-clip system. (SH)

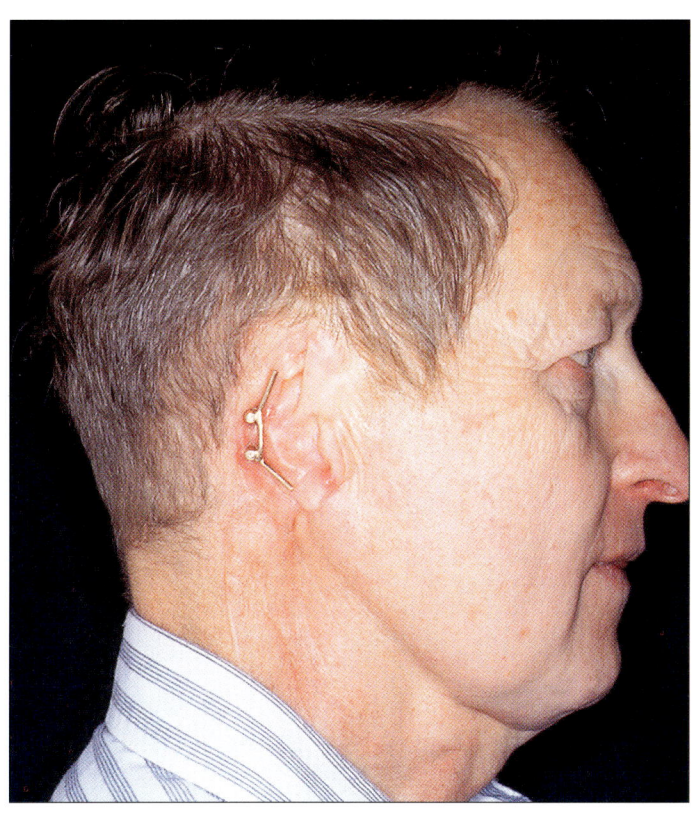

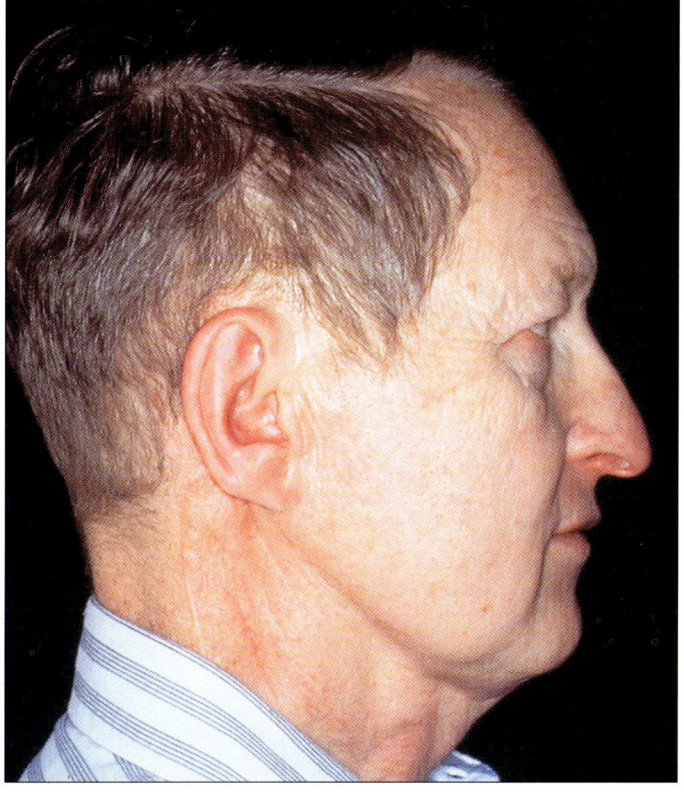

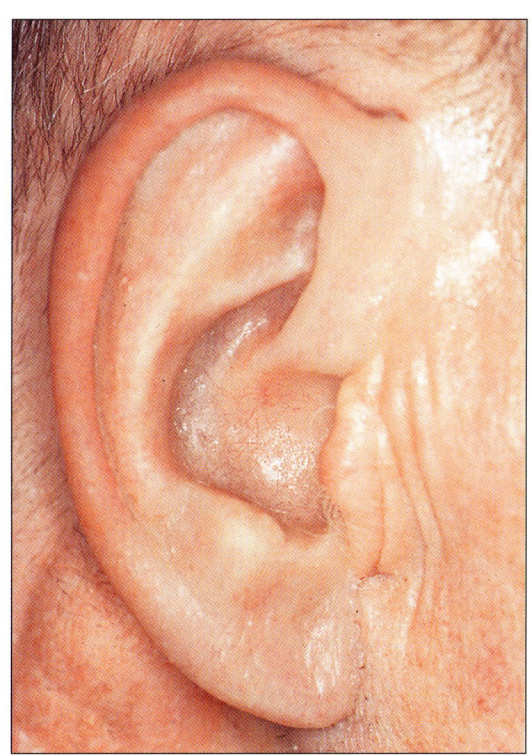

PATIENT PRESENTATION 15

15 *This man underwent a right auriculectomy due to a malignant melanoma in 1991. After the operation, he was informed about a bone-anchored auricular prosthesis, but he decided against it. He later changed his mind. A two-stage procedure was performed, with two fixtures placed in the mastoid process. About 3 weeks after the abutment connection (March 1994), he was fitted with a silicone auricular prosthesis. (KB)*

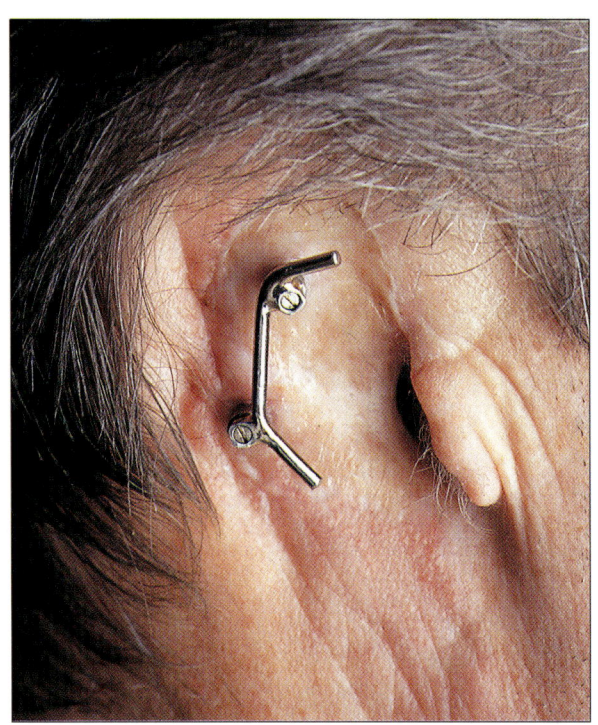
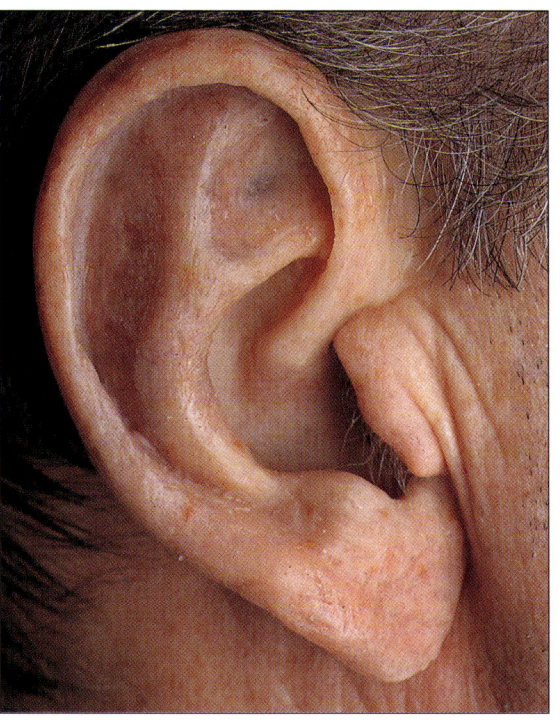
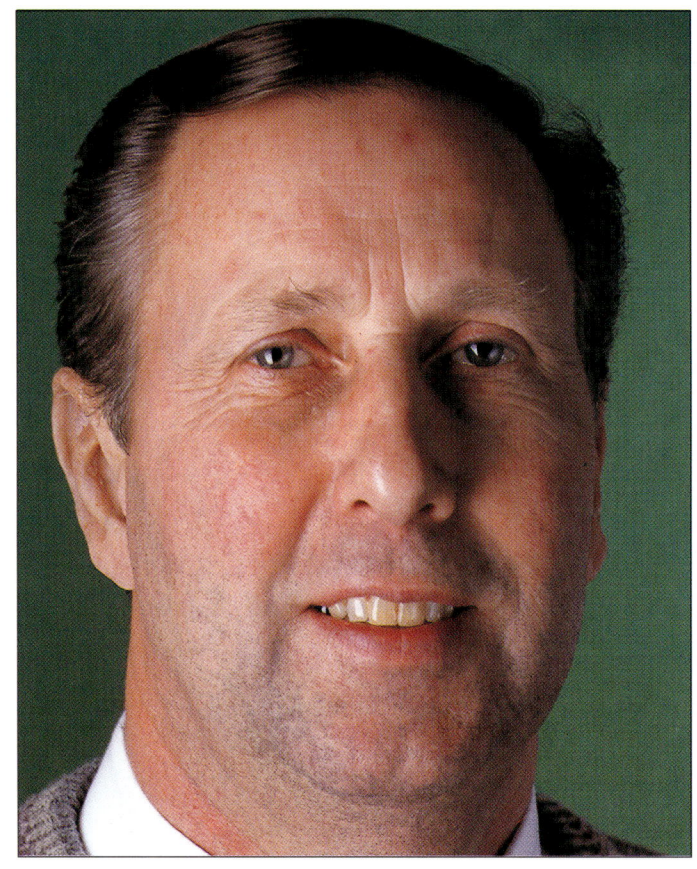

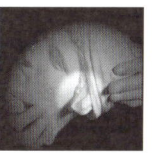

16 *This 24-year-old man suffered a traumatic avulsion of his right ear in a motor vehicle accident in 1986. He decided to have a bone-anchored prosthesis. In 1992, two fixtures were placed in the mastoid area, and 6 months later, abutments were connected. After the healing period, a silicone auricular prosthesis was retained with a bar-and-clip system. (SG)*

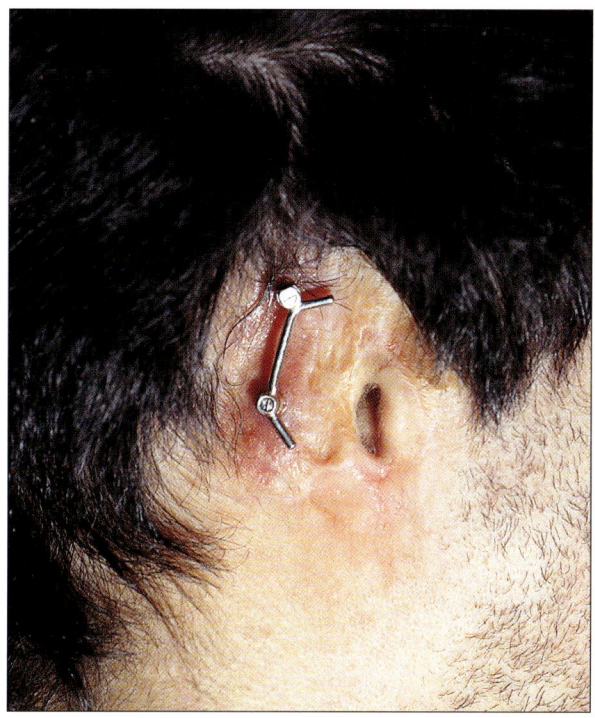
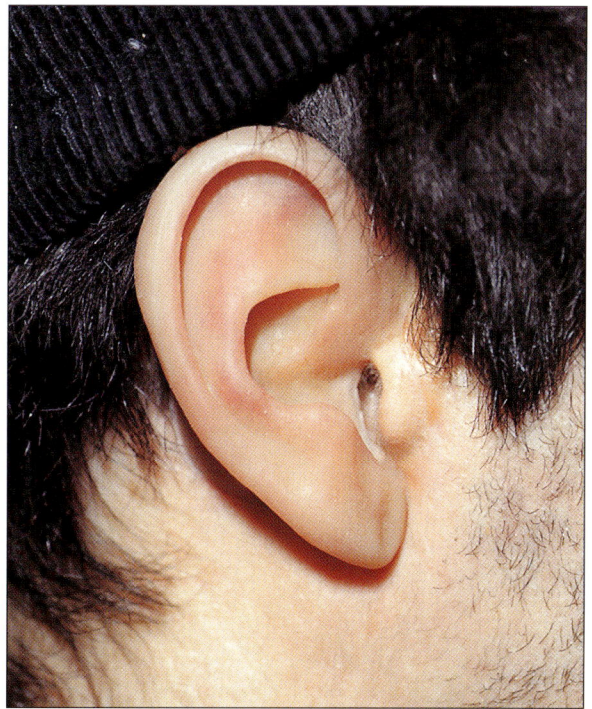
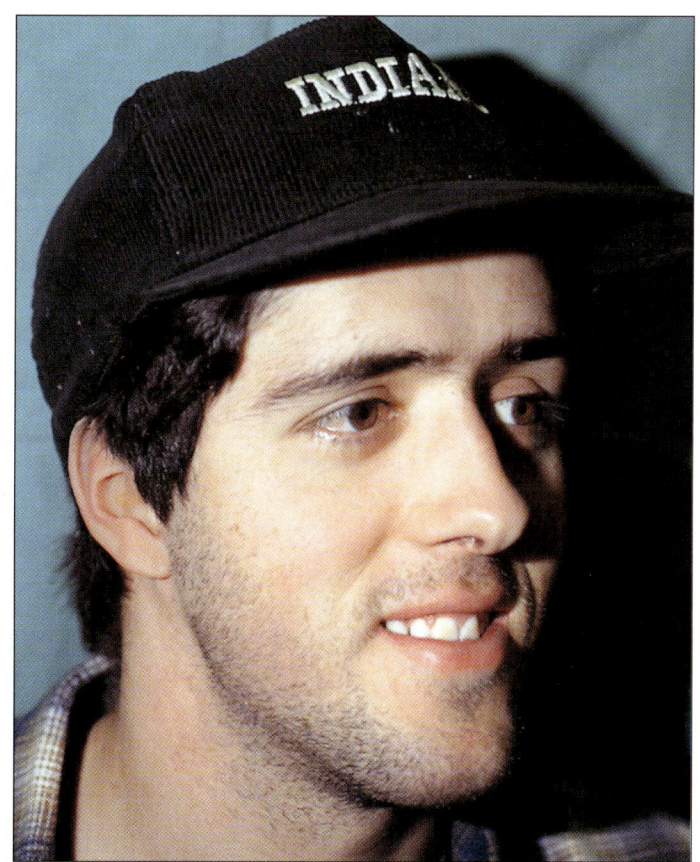

Patient Presentation 17

17 *This 54-year-old man underwent a right auriculectomy due to a squamous cell carcinoma. A two-stage procedure was performed and three fixtures were placed to retain the prosthesis on a bar-and-clip system. After the healing period, a silicone auricular prosthesis was fitted. (SG)*

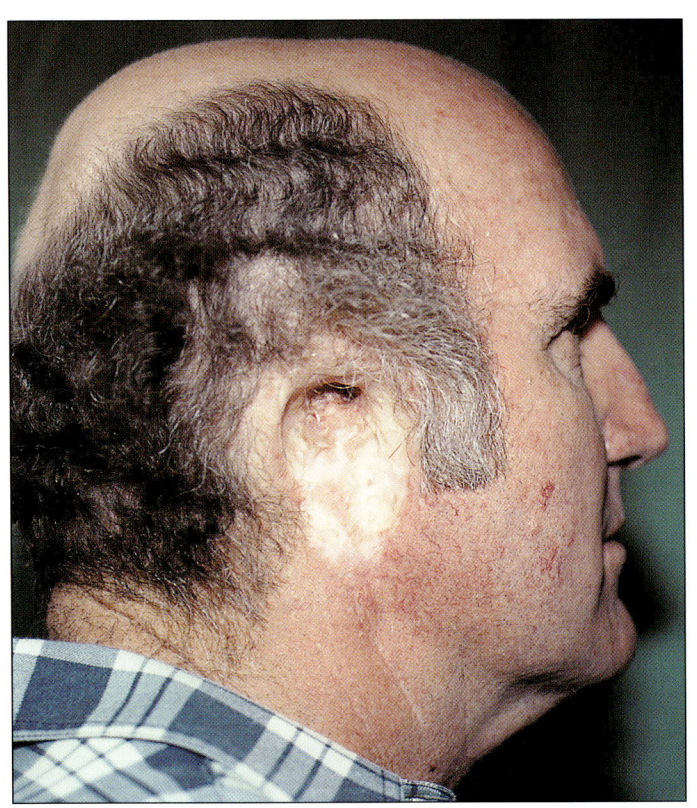
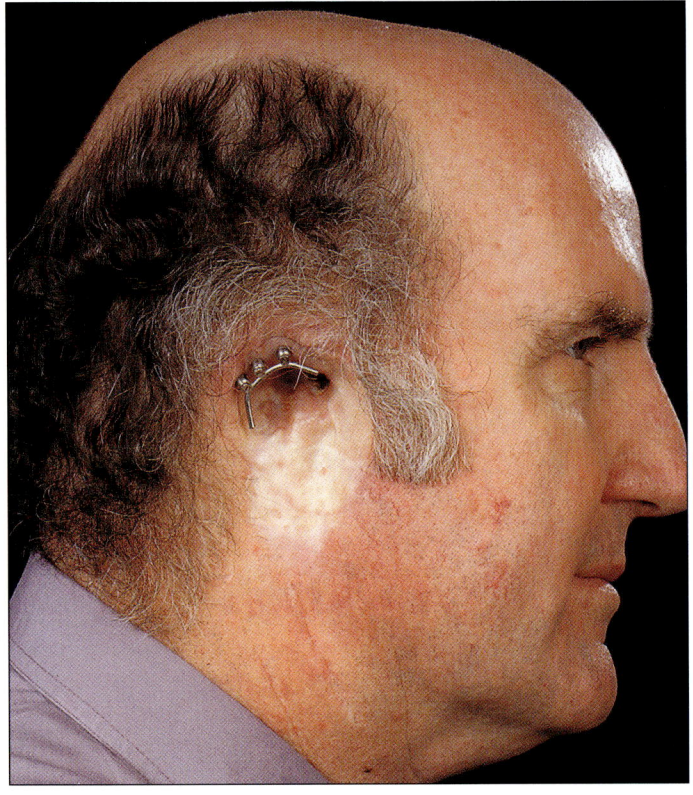
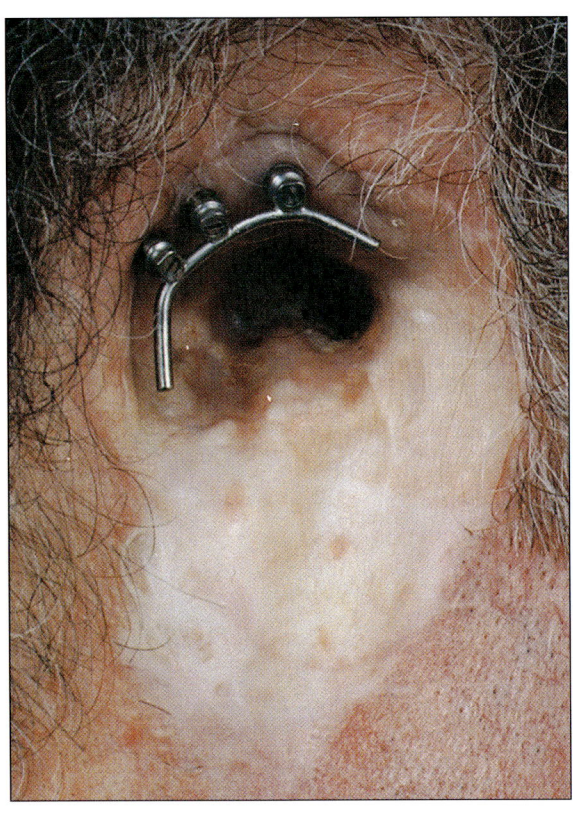
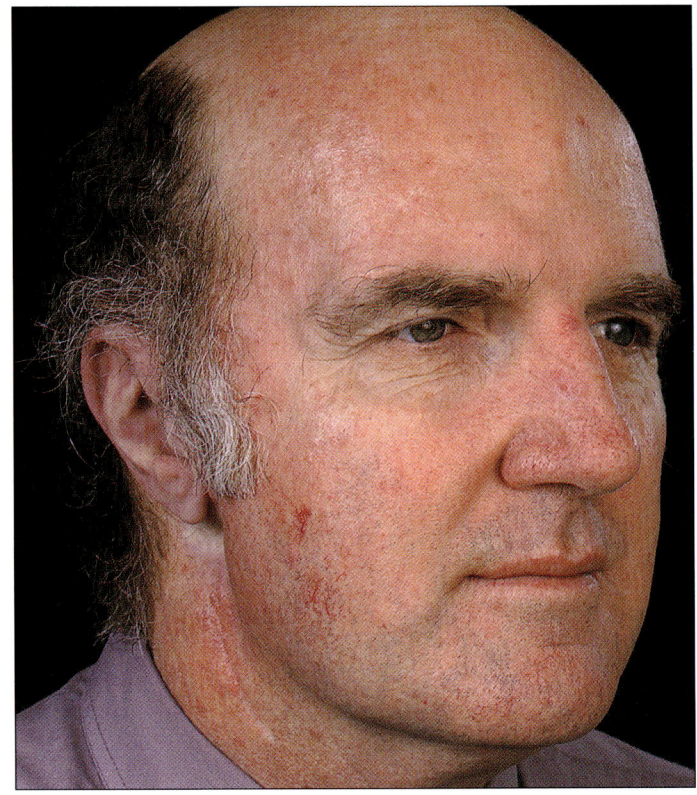

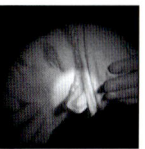

18 *This young man was born with right hemifacial microsomia. He decided to undergo osseointegrated prosthetic reconstruction, and two craniofacial fixtures were placed in the mastoid area. At a later stage, abutments were connected, and after the healing period, a silicone auricular prosthesis was fitted. Retention was achieved with a bar-and-clip system. (DM)*

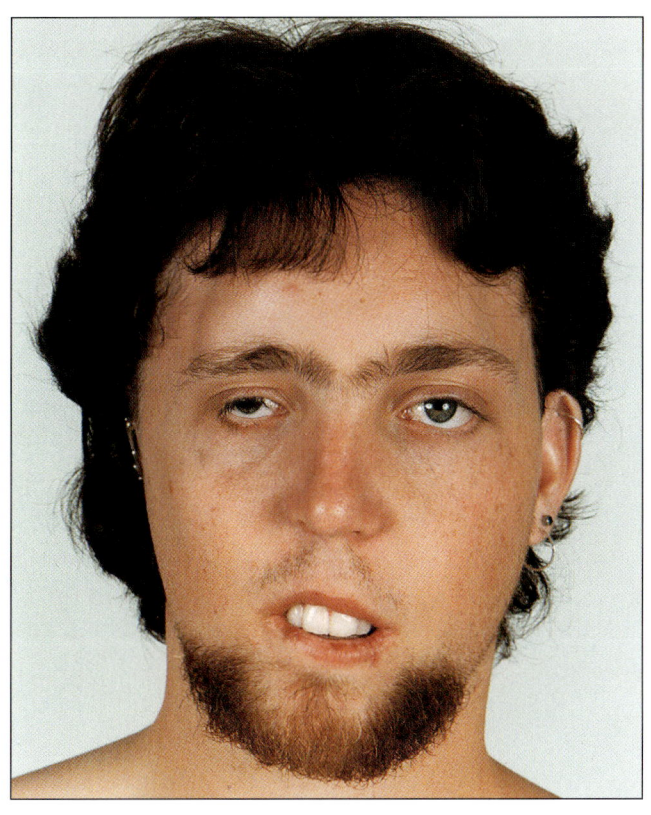
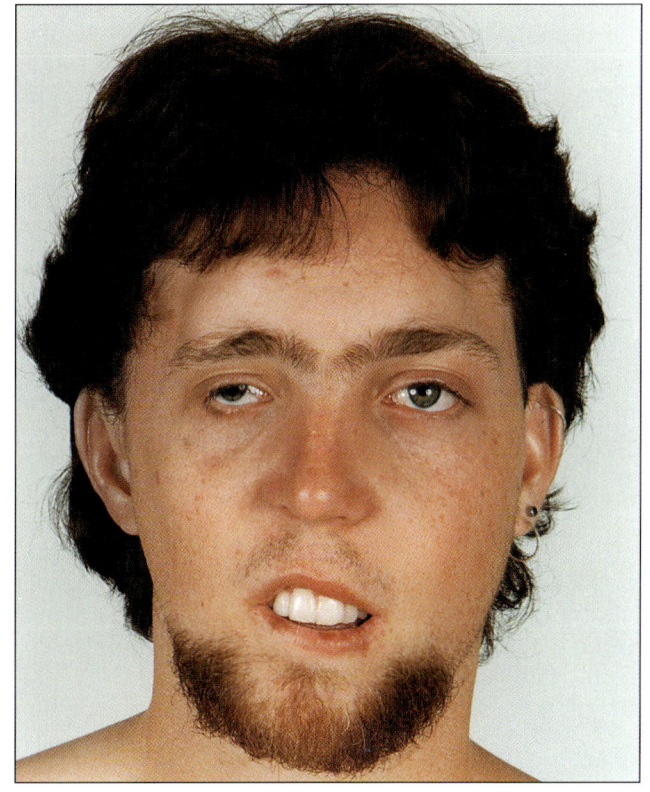
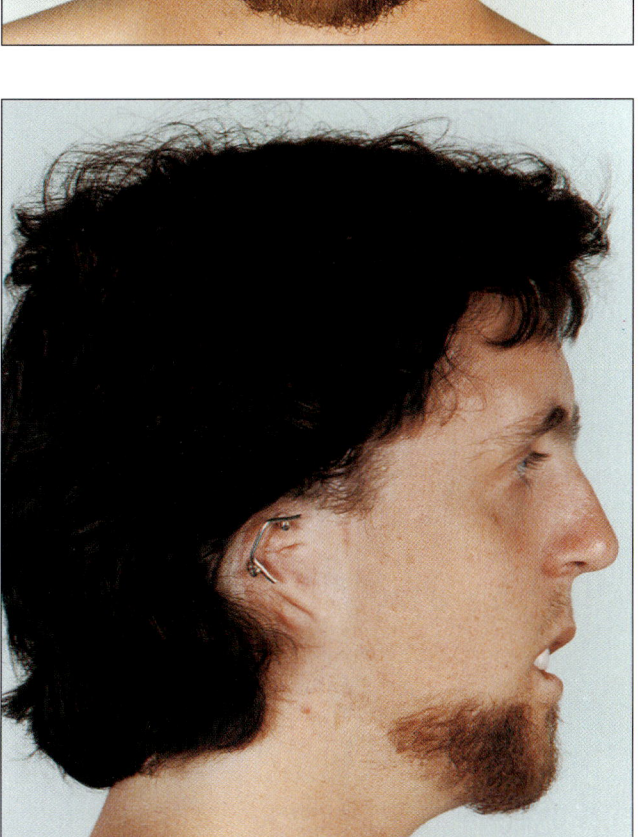
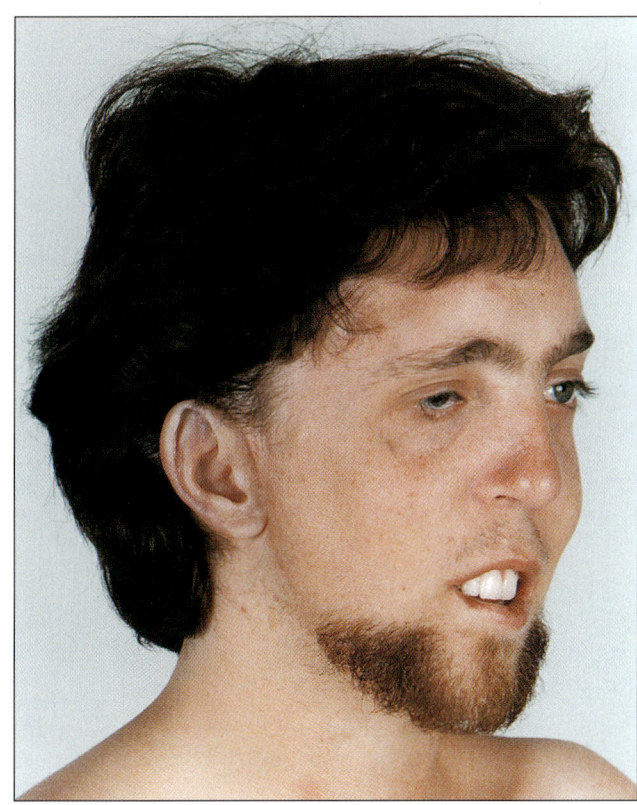

19 *This 31-year-old man was born with a deformity of the right auricle and absence of the auditory canal. In 1968, surgical reorganization of the tissues of his ear was attempted and in 1969 he had a silicone implant that was removed 1 year later, at which time he had a cartilage graft from the seventh right rib. He was seen in 1982 and no further surgery was advised. In October 1995, a silicone auricular prosthesis was anchored on two osseointegrated fixtures. (IM)*

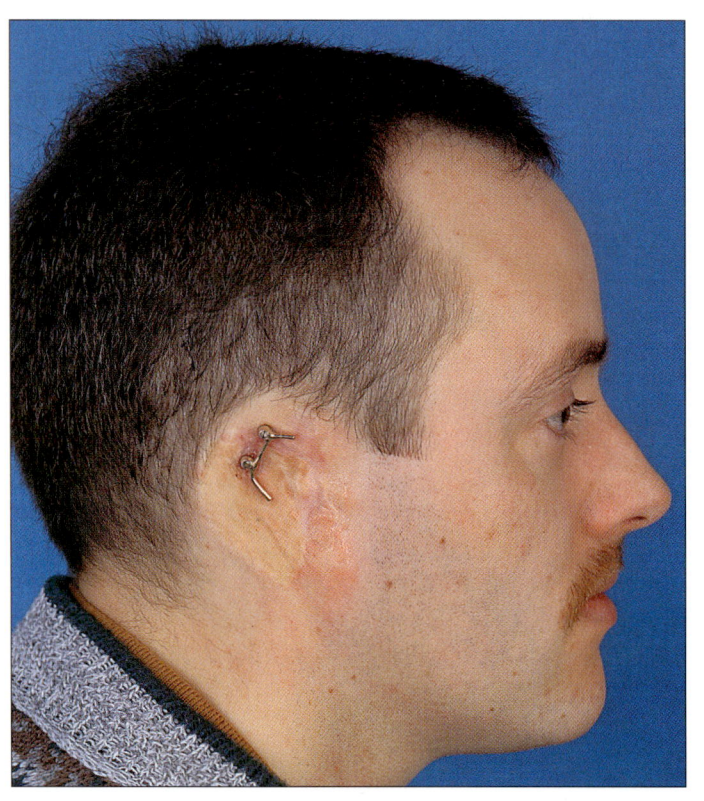
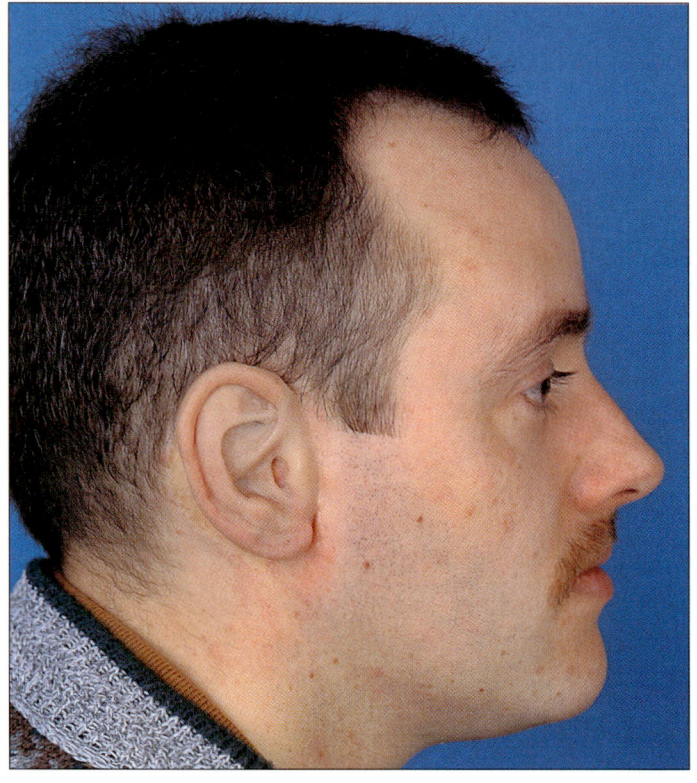
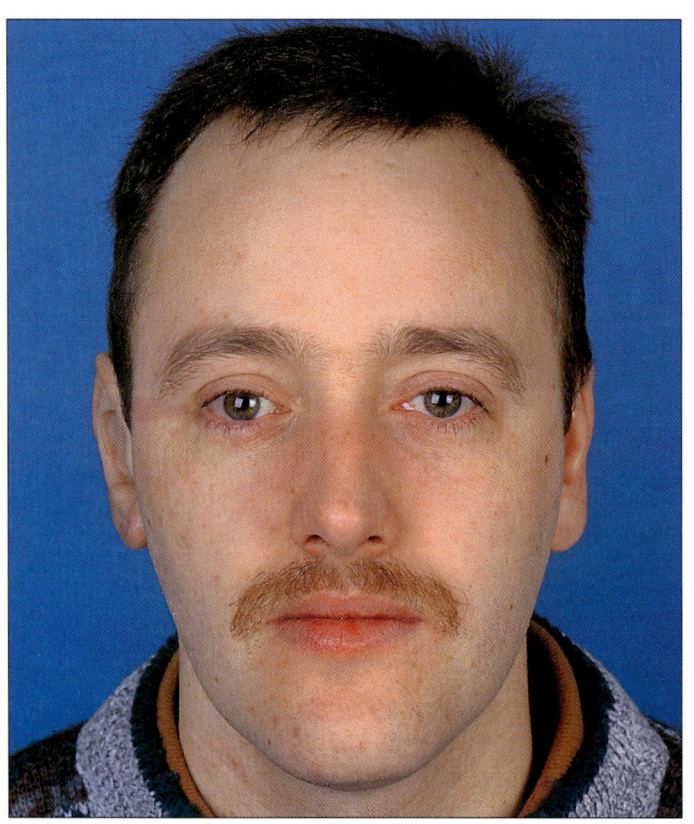
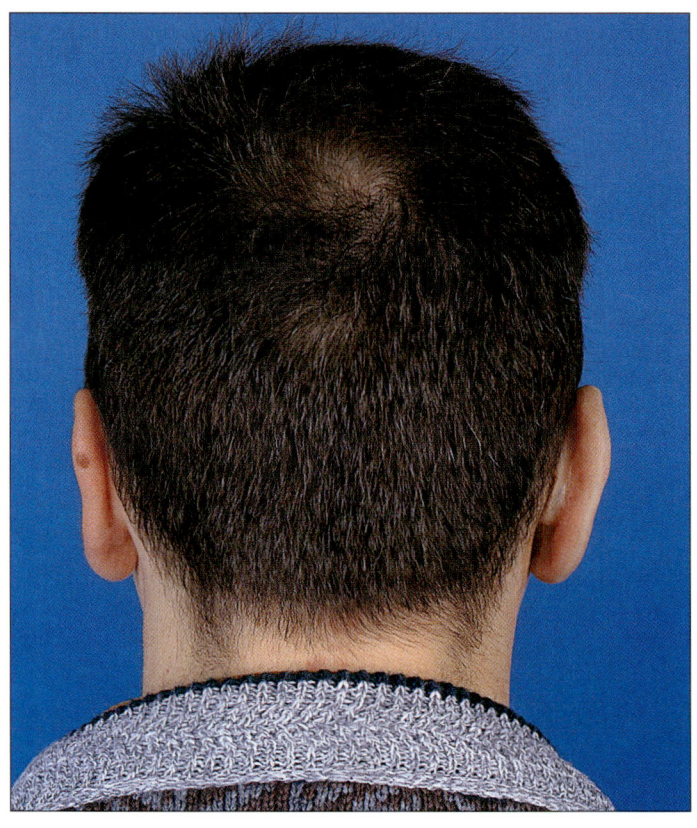

20 *This 25-year-old woman had a right auricular amputation as a result of an automobile accident. Rehabilitation was achieved by fabricating a silicone prosthesis mechanically retained with a bar-and-clip system, connected onto two osseointegrated fixtures. If because of bone density or craniofacial anomalies the implants cannot be placed in the optimal site, the acrylic plate may extend beyond the pinna from the lateral and posterolateral views, which would be esthetically unacceptable. For this patient, the space between the tragus and antitragus was widened and the rostral attachment of the helix was moved to conceal the fact that the entire ear was moved posteriorly. (GD)*

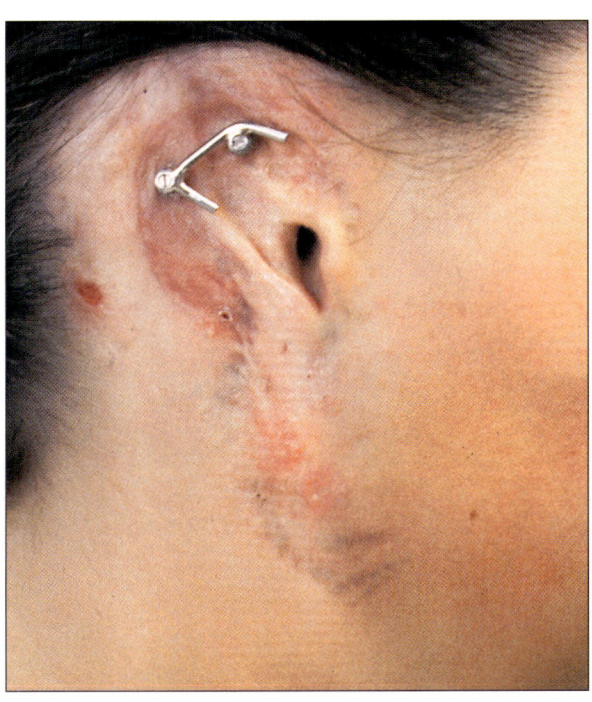
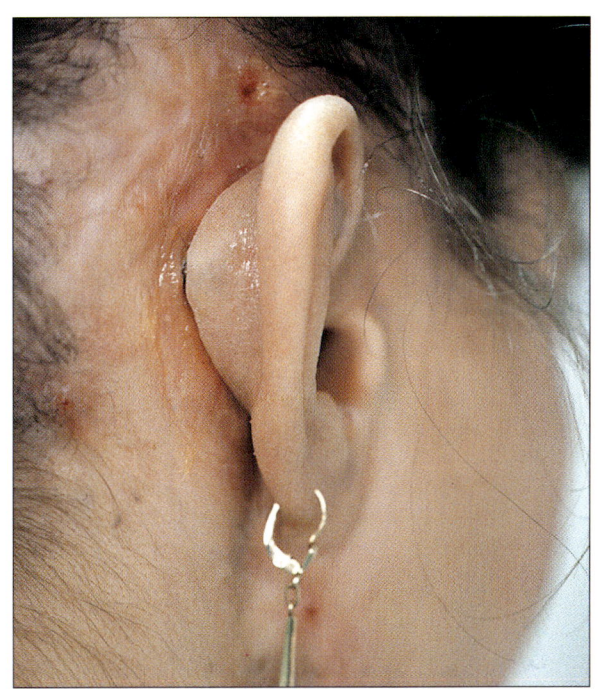
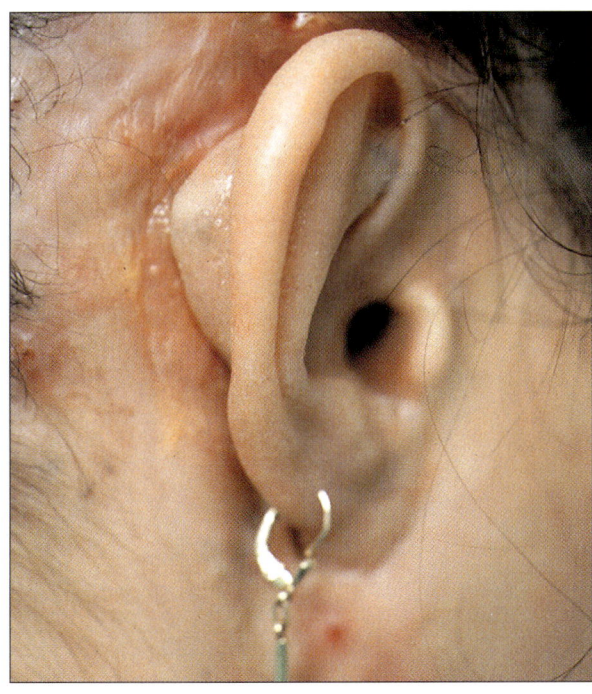
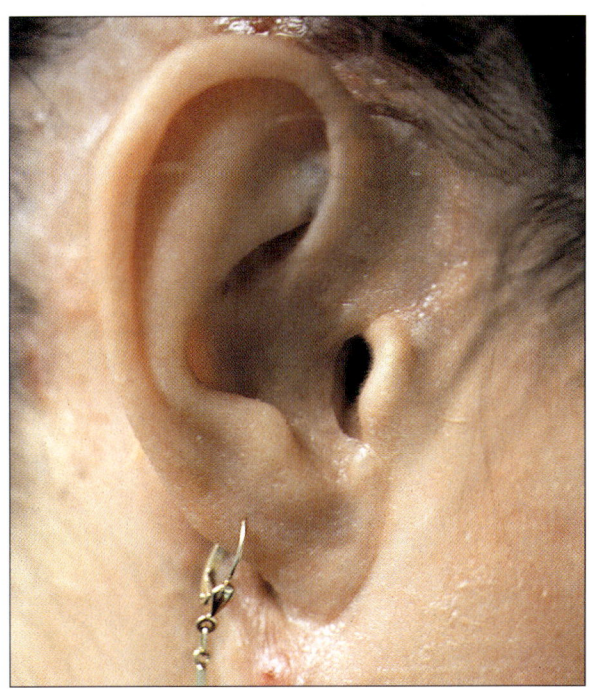

Nasal Defects

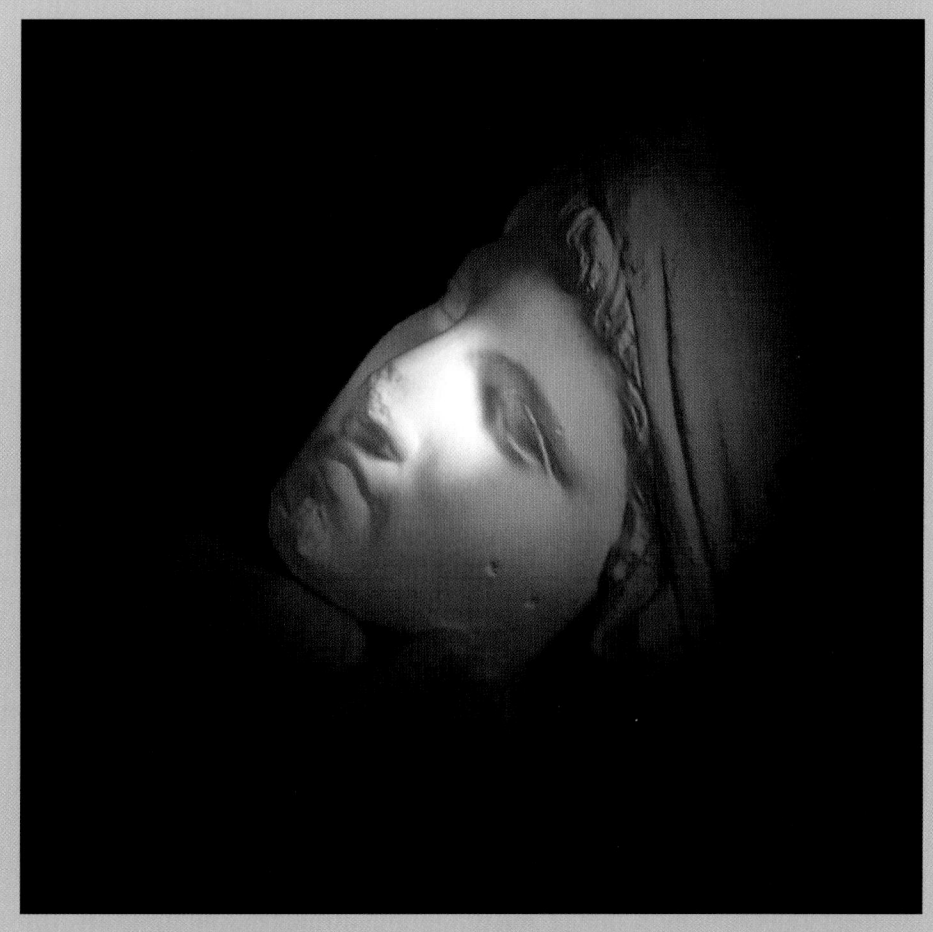

Patient Presentation 1

1 This 14-year-old boy underwent a total rhinectomy and postoperative chemotherapy due to a rhabdomyosarcoma at the age of 5. He was provided with an immediate adhesive-retained temporary prosthesis. After the healing period, a new nasal prosthesis was fabricated. To accommodate facial growth, the prosthesis was replaced at least once a year. It is anticipated that this patient will undergo surgical reconstruction of his nose before going to college. (AF)

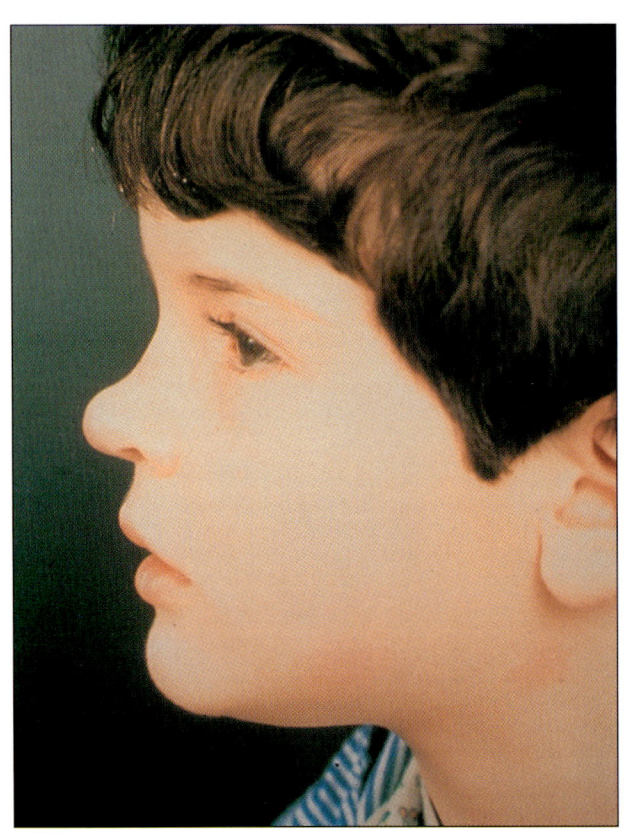

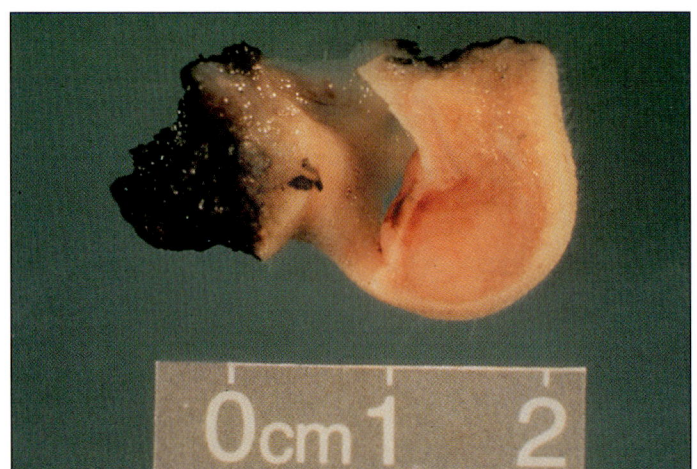

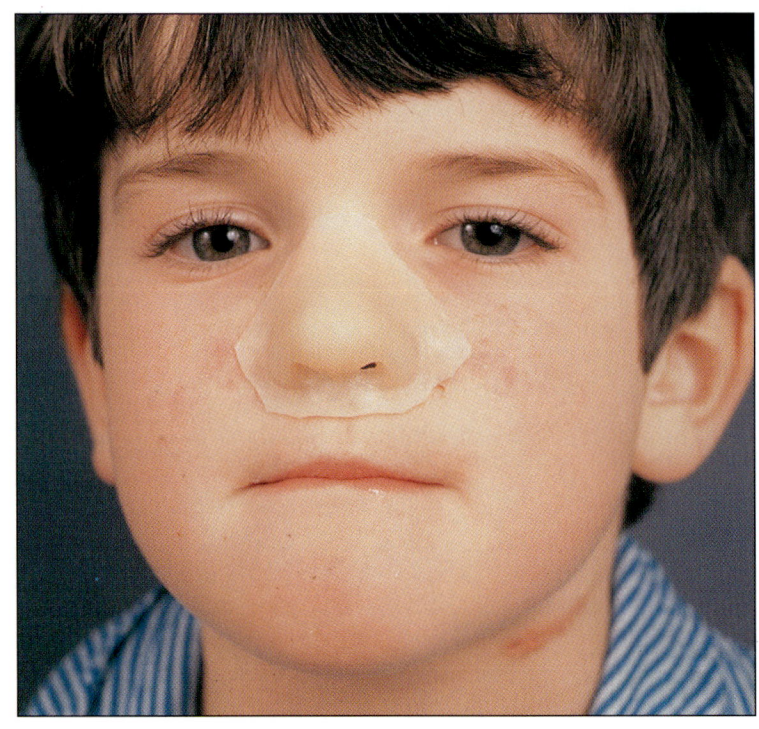

PATIENT PRESENTATION 1

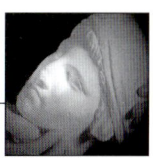
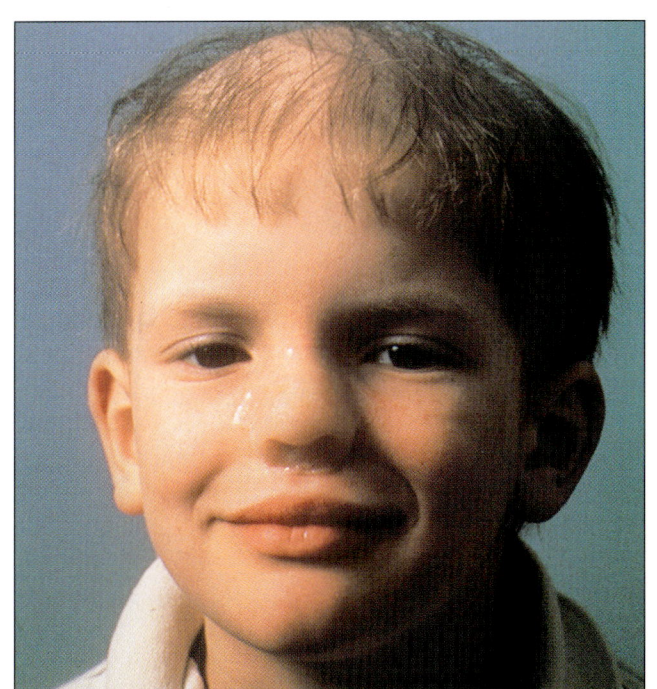
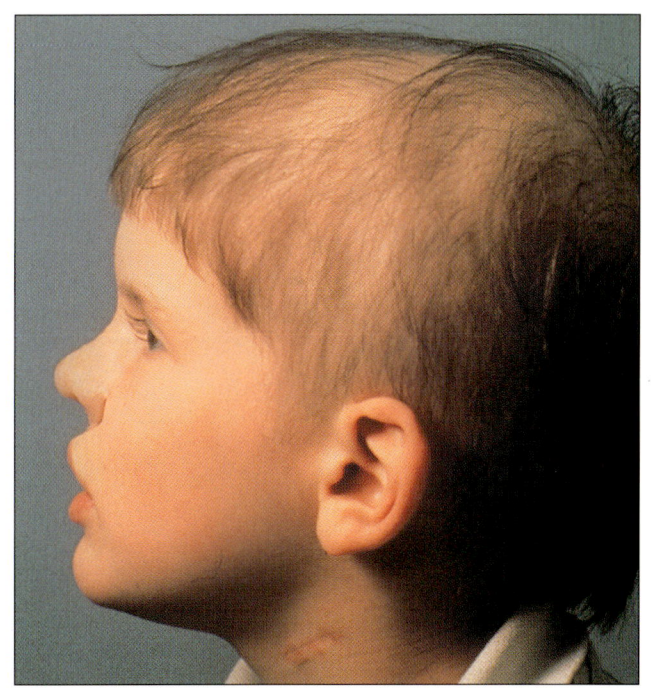
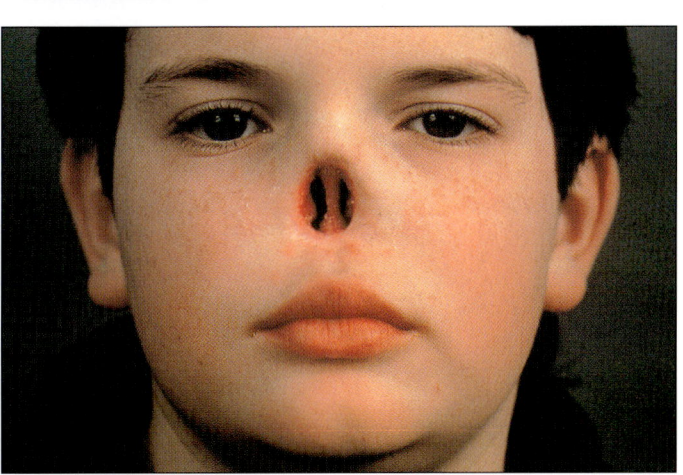
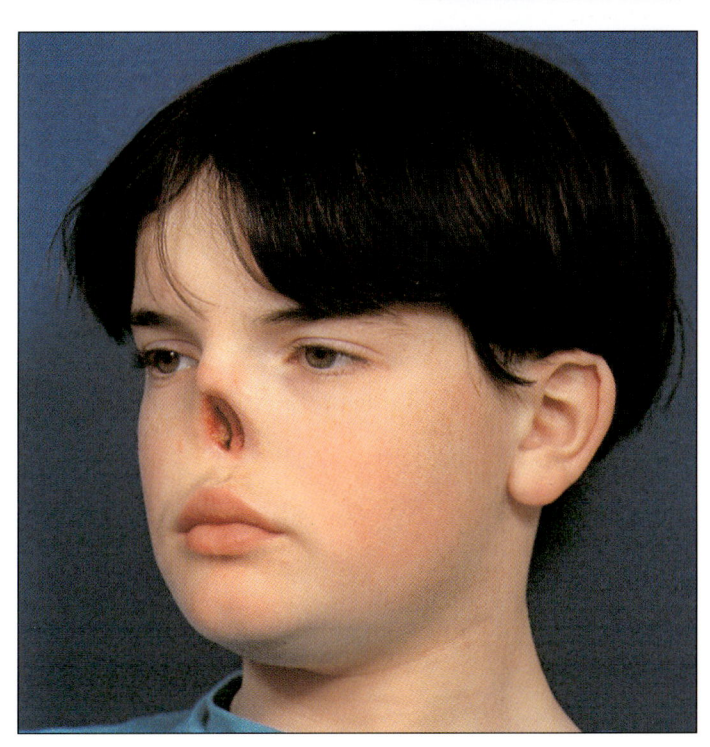
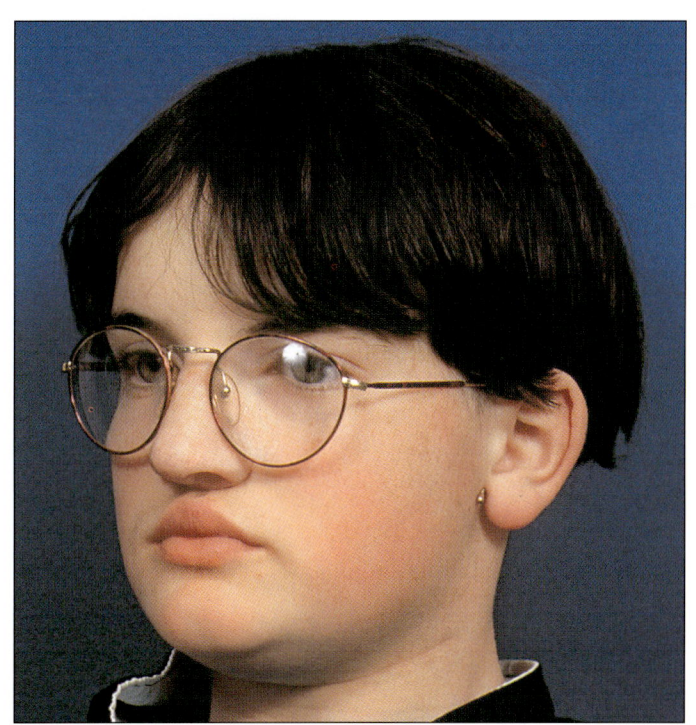

PATIENT PRESENTATION 2

2 This 74-year-old man underwent a partial rhinectomy and anterior and medial left maxillectomy due to a malignant neurofibrosarcoma. He also underwent radiation therapy and chemotherapy. When the soft tissue healed, an adhesive-retained silicone partial nasal prosthesis was fitted, restoring the missing facial structure. (AF)

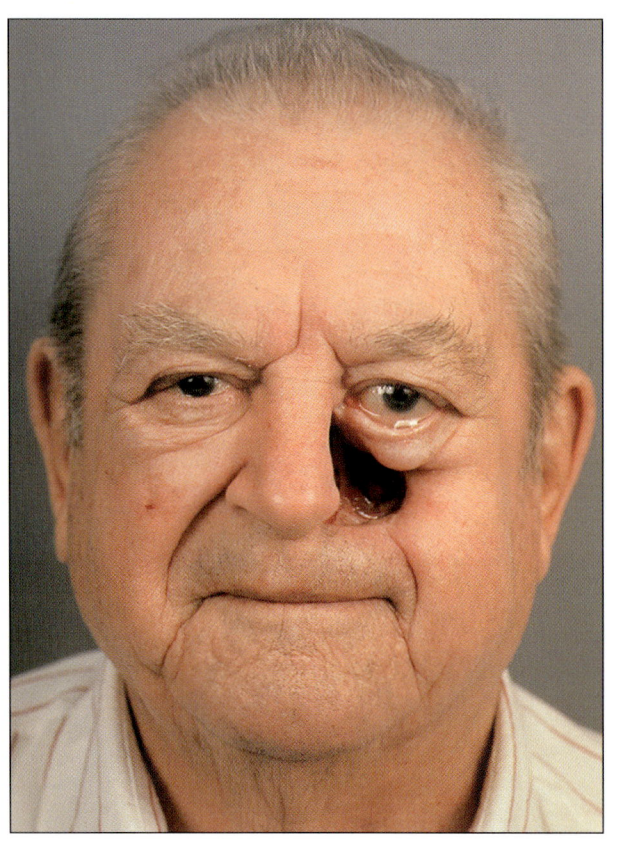
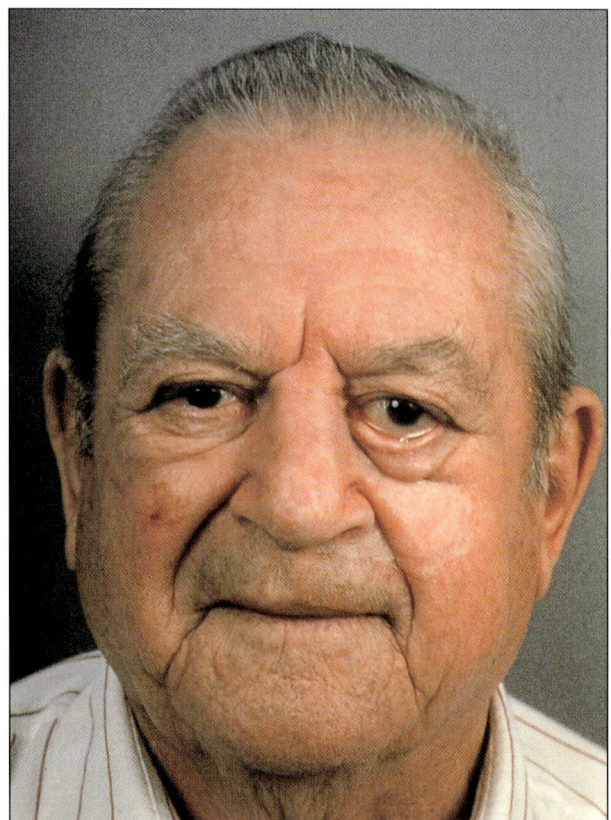
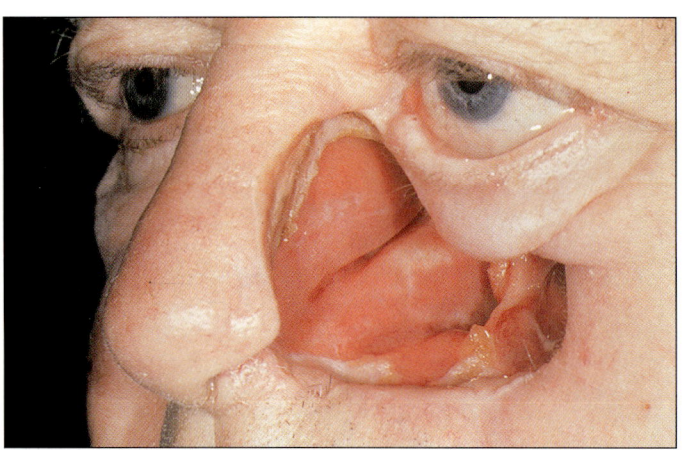
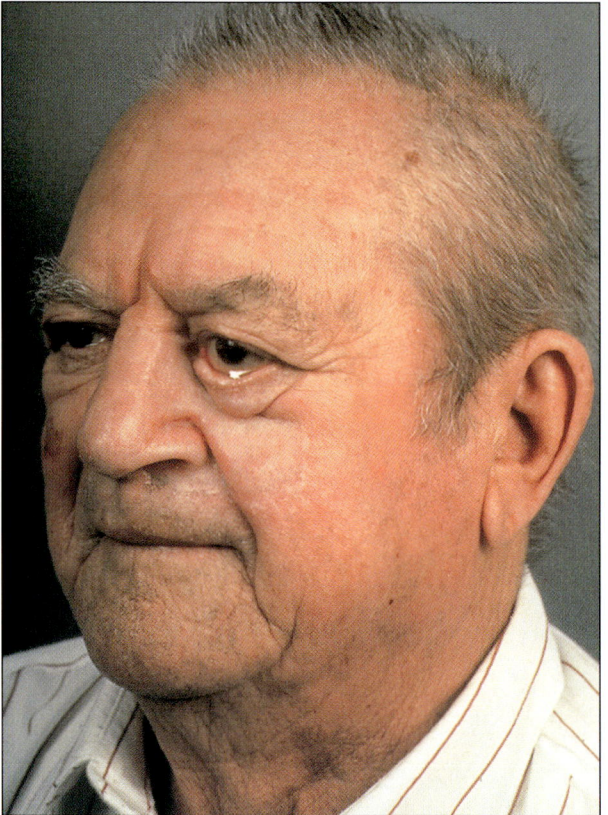

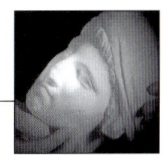

PATIENT PRESENTATION 3

3 *This 71-year-old man underwent a right alar excision due to a squamous cell carcinoma. An interim adhesive-retained silicone prosthesis was provided for the patient, followed by alar reconstruction. (AF)*

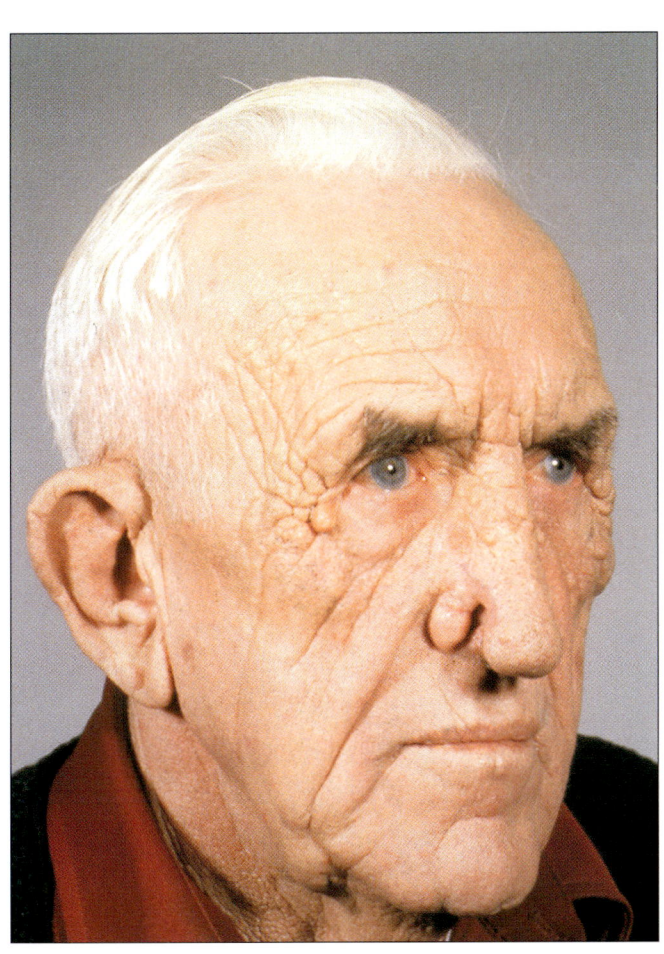

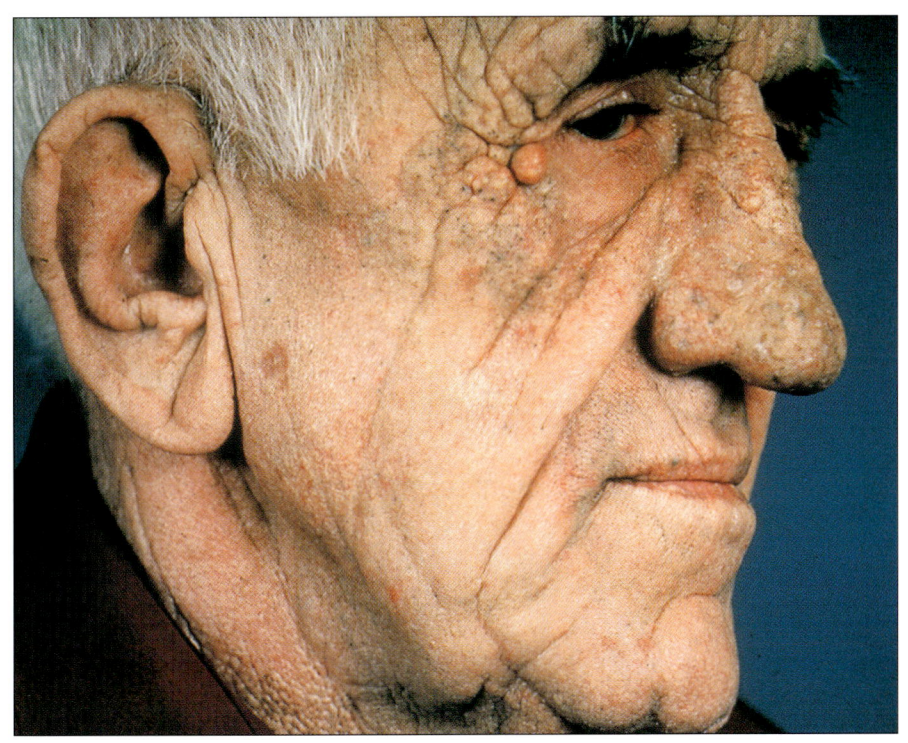

Patient Presentation 4

4 *This 70-year-old man underwent a total rhinectomy due to a basal cell carcinoma. As part of the treatment, he received radiation therapy and chemotherapy. After the healing period, he was provided with an adhesive-retained silicone nasal prosthesis. (AF)*

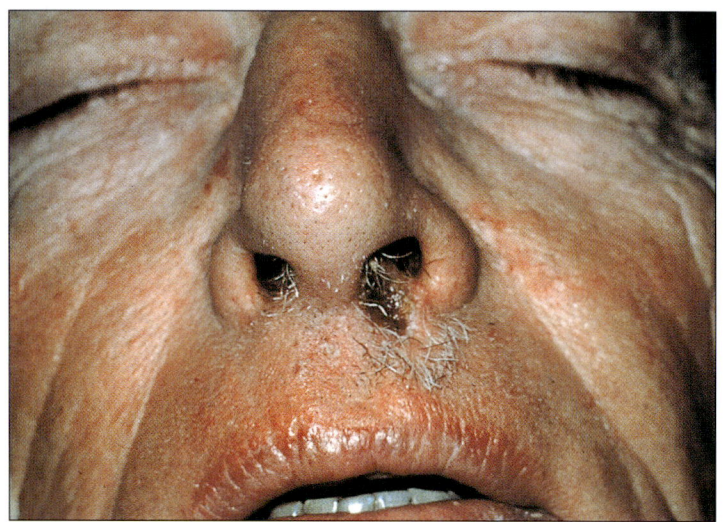
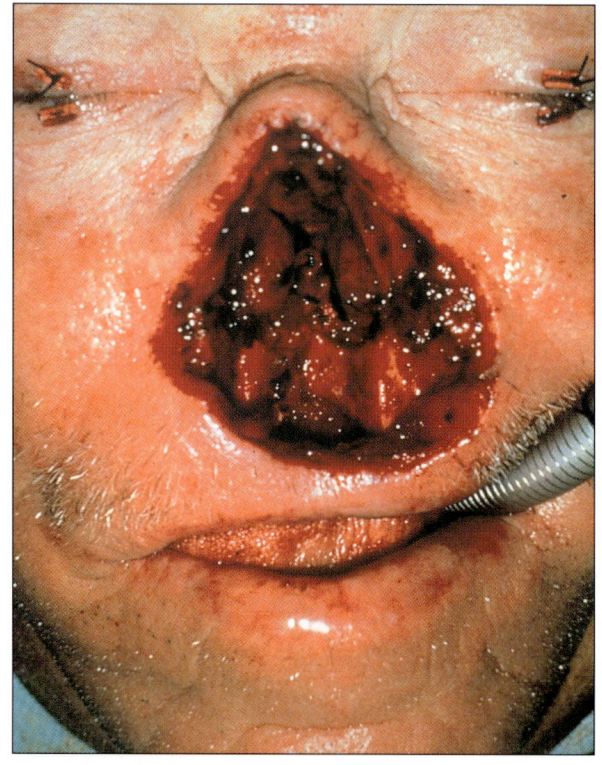
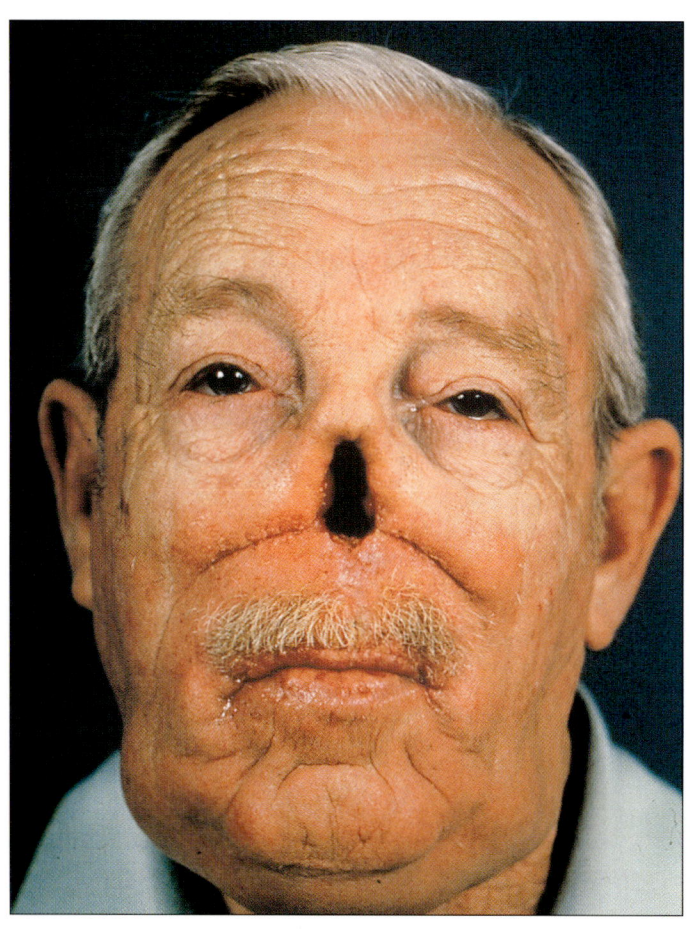
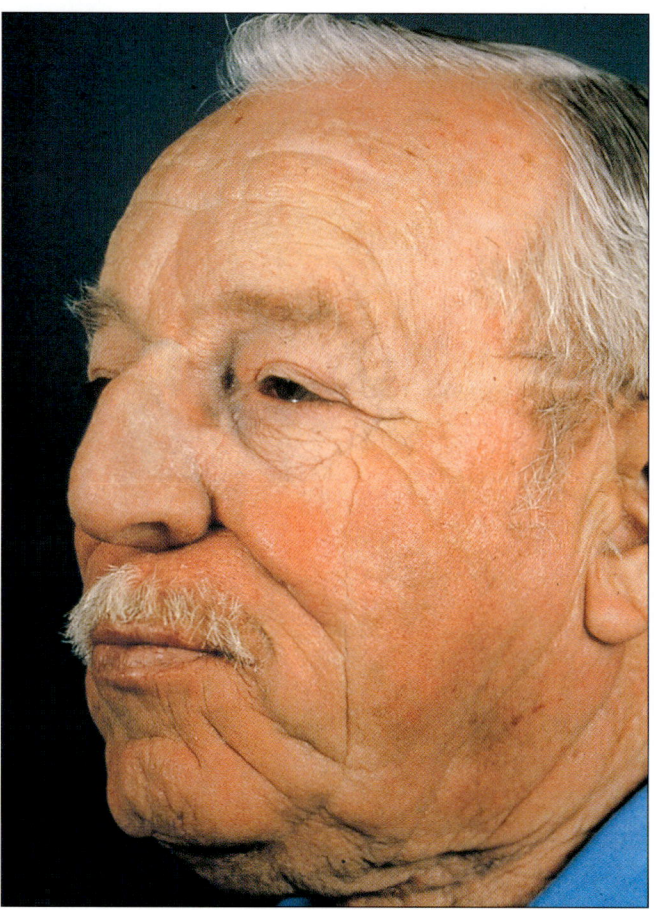

PATIENT PRESENTATION 5

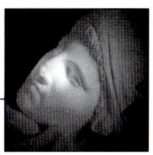

5 *This 66-year-old man underwent a rhinectomy due to squamous cell carcinoma. The acrylic and silicone nasal prosthesis was magnetically retained to the superior surface of the patient's obturator by an intermediate piece, which in turn was magnetically retained to both the nasal prosthesis and the intraoral obturator. (GG)*

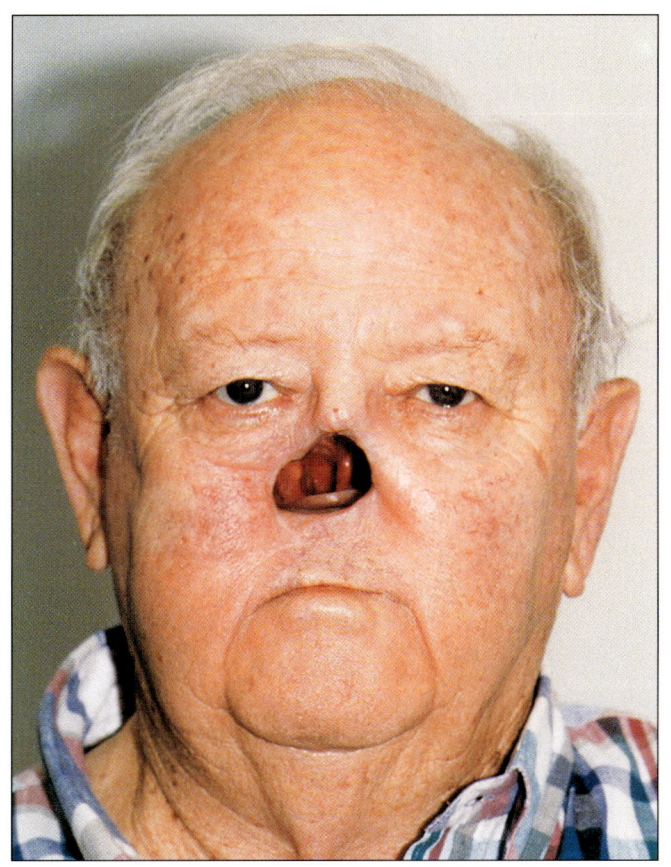
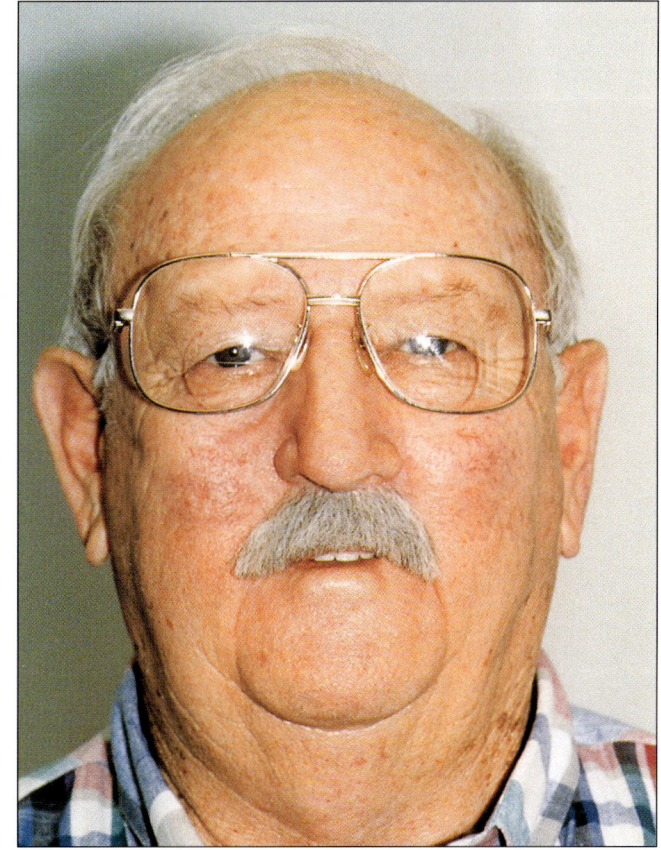
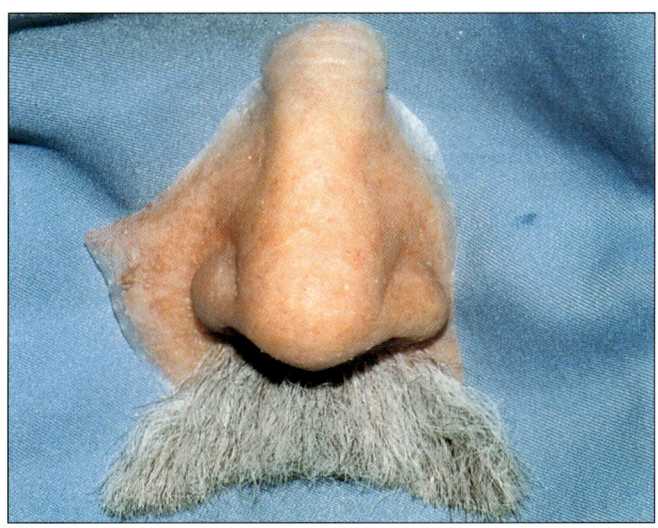
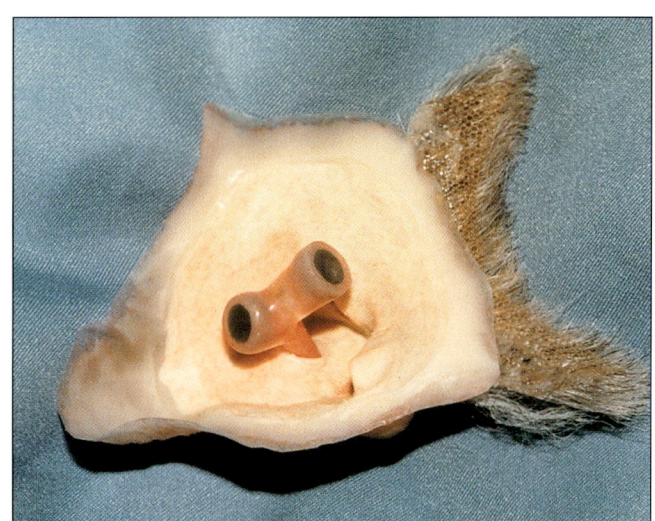

6 *This 83-year-old woman underwent a nasal resection due to basal cell carcinoma. She did not receive radiation therapy, and after the healing period two fixtures were placed into the nasal floor. A framework was fabricated, splinting the implants, and two magnets were used to retain the nasal prosthesis. (DT)*

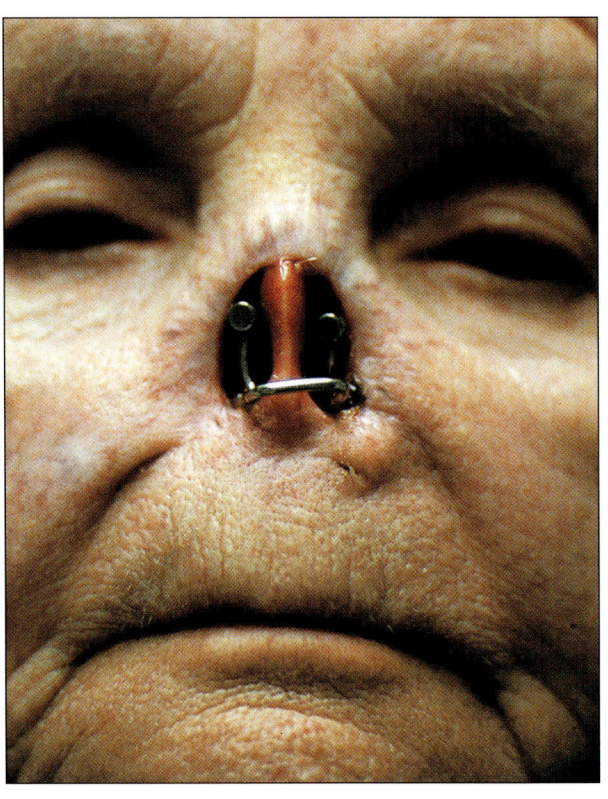
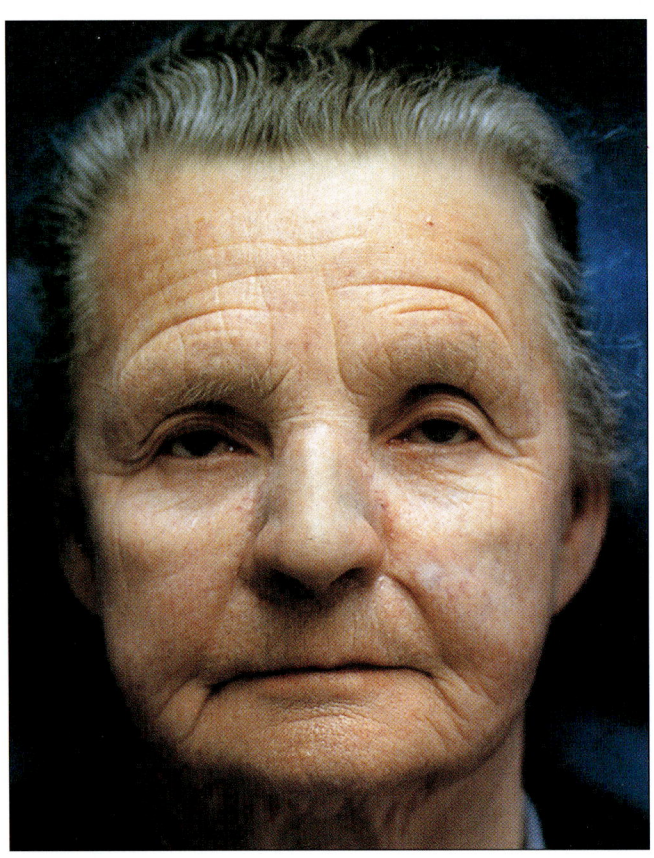
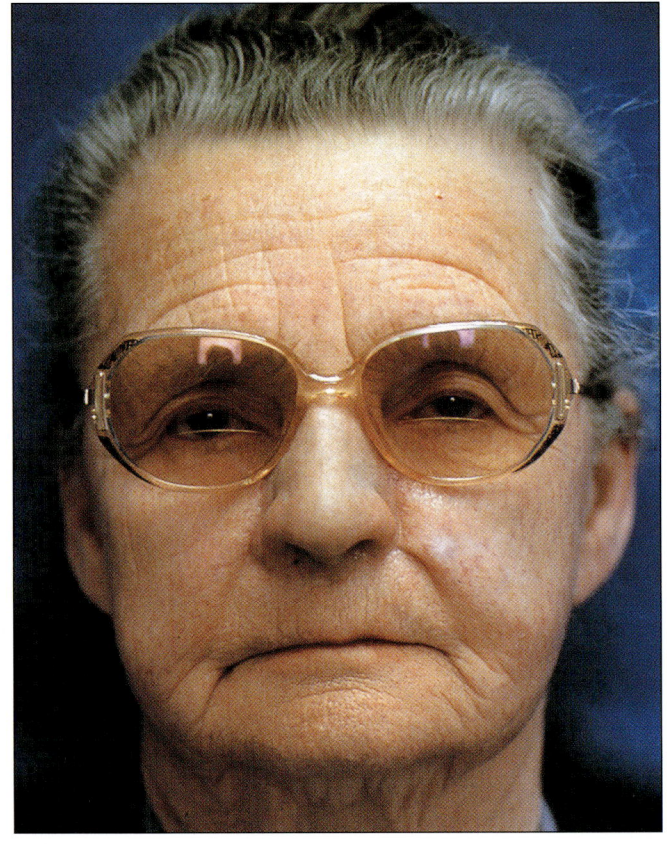

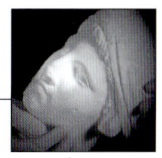

7 This 70-year-old woman underwent an extensive nasal resection due to recurrent squamous cell carcinoma involving the nasal tip, septum, and the right cheek, at the age of 62. Two fixtures were placed in the maxillary bone. The fixture placed on the left side failed to osseointegrate, and a new one was placed to the right of it. A gold bar was fabricated to splint the two fixtures so that a silicone nasal prosthesis could be mechanically retained to it by gold clips. (IH)

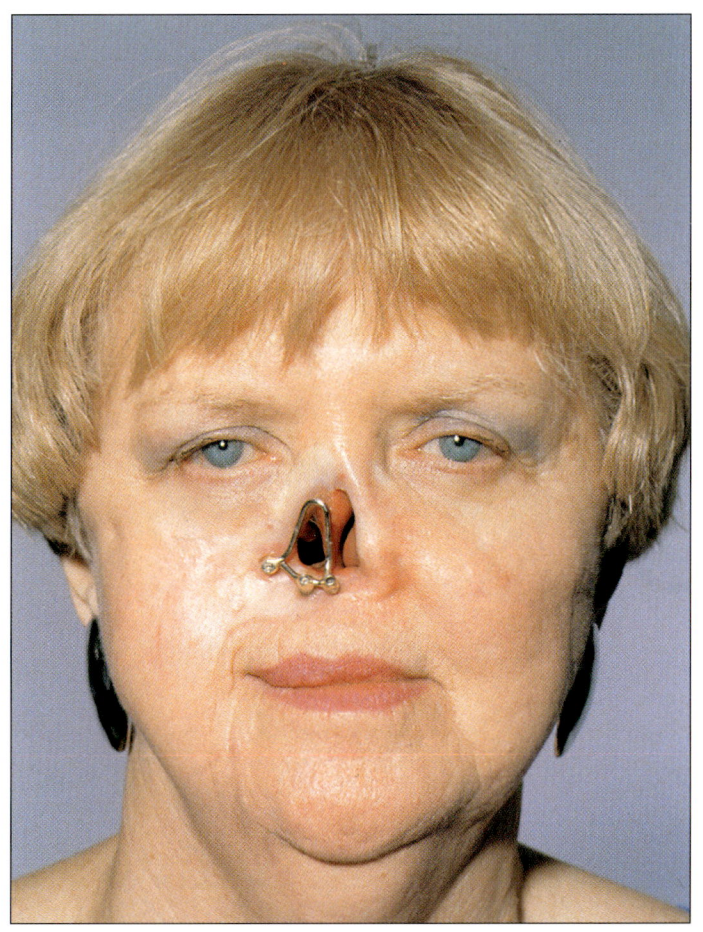
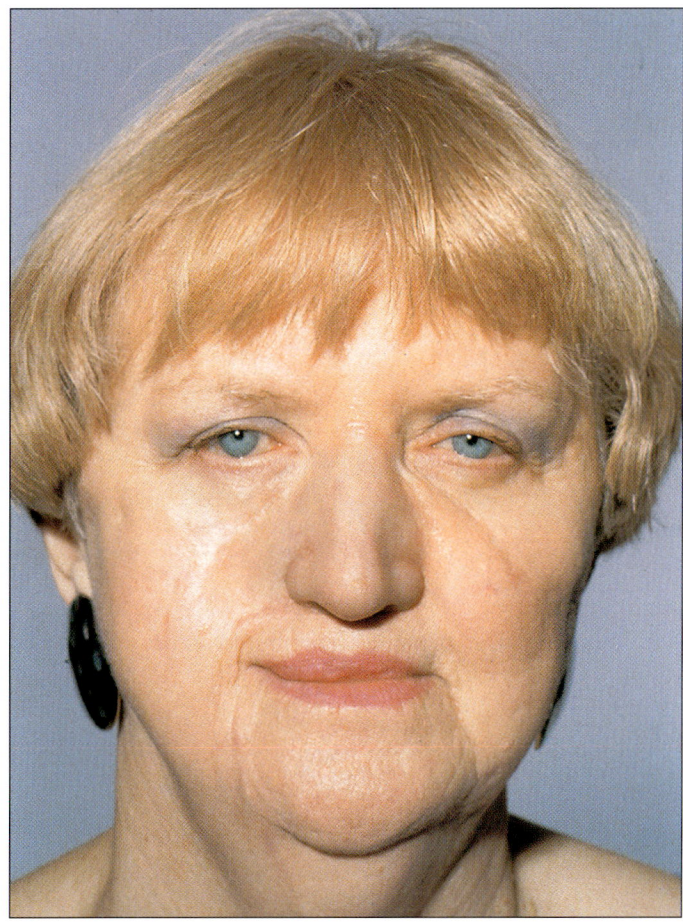

(continued)

PATIENT PRESENTATION 7

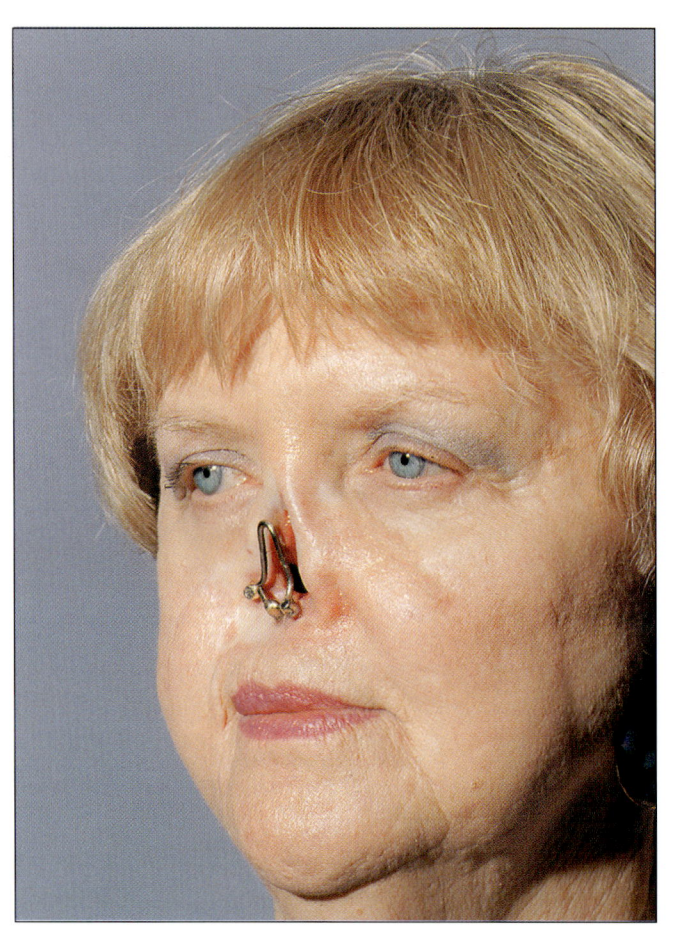
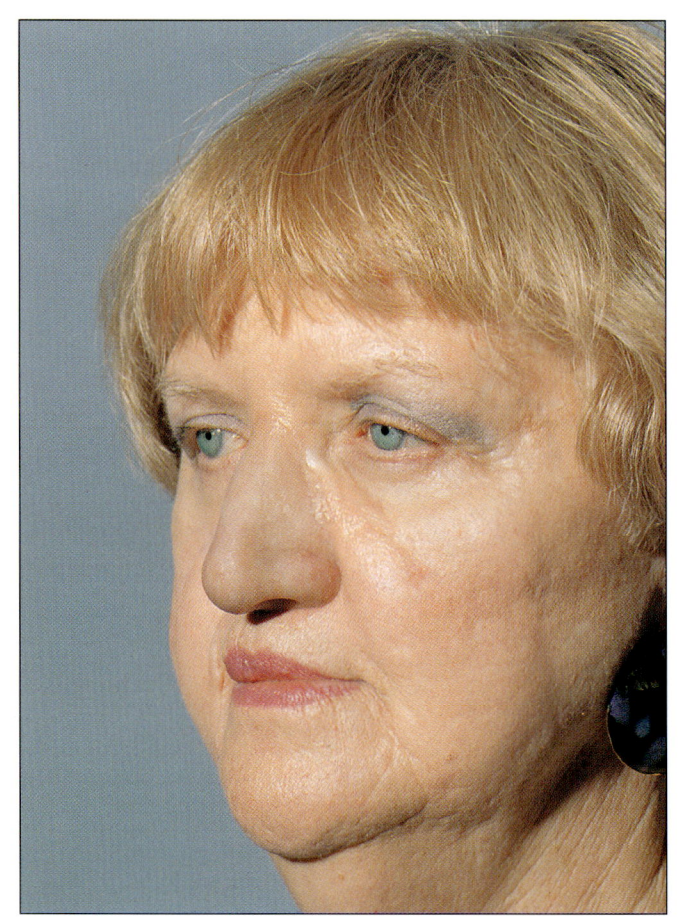
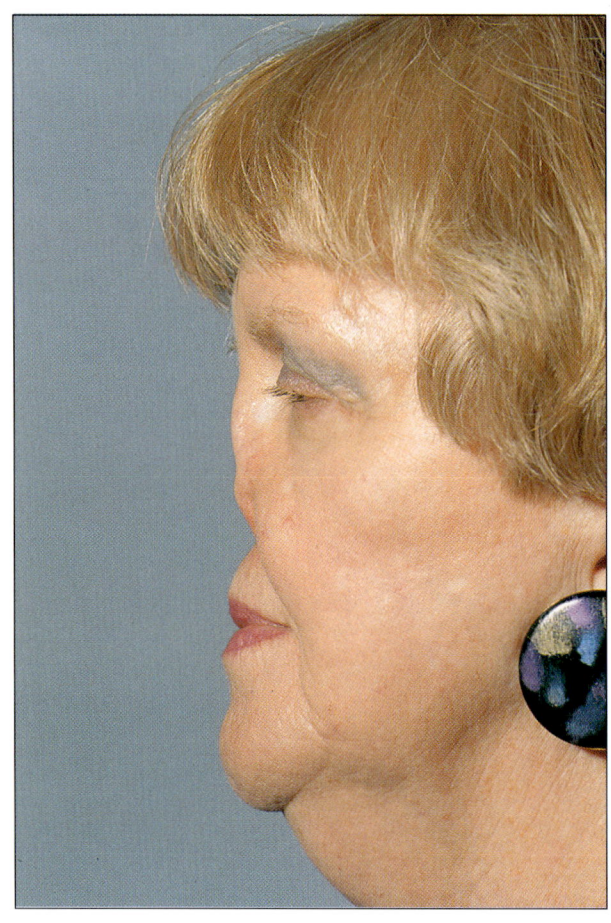
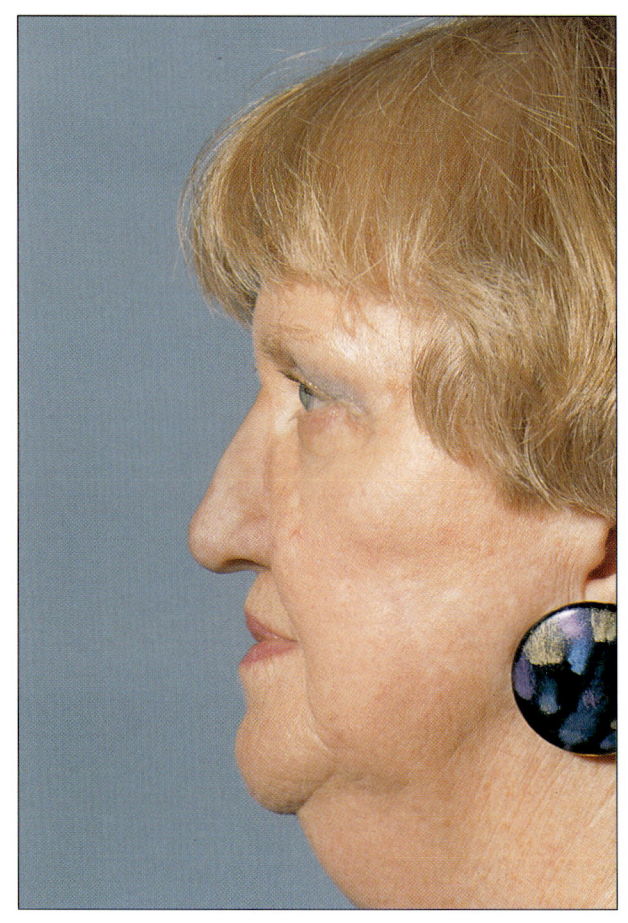

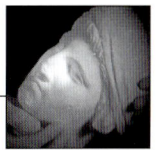

8 *This 80-year-old woman underwent a total rhinectomy due to squamous cell carcinoma of the nasal septum. Two years later, three fixtures were placed, but the one placed on the left side failed to osseointegrate. After the abutment connection, a framework was fabricated splinting the fixtures, and the silicone and acrylic bone-anchored nasal prosthesis was retained with magnets. (SH)*

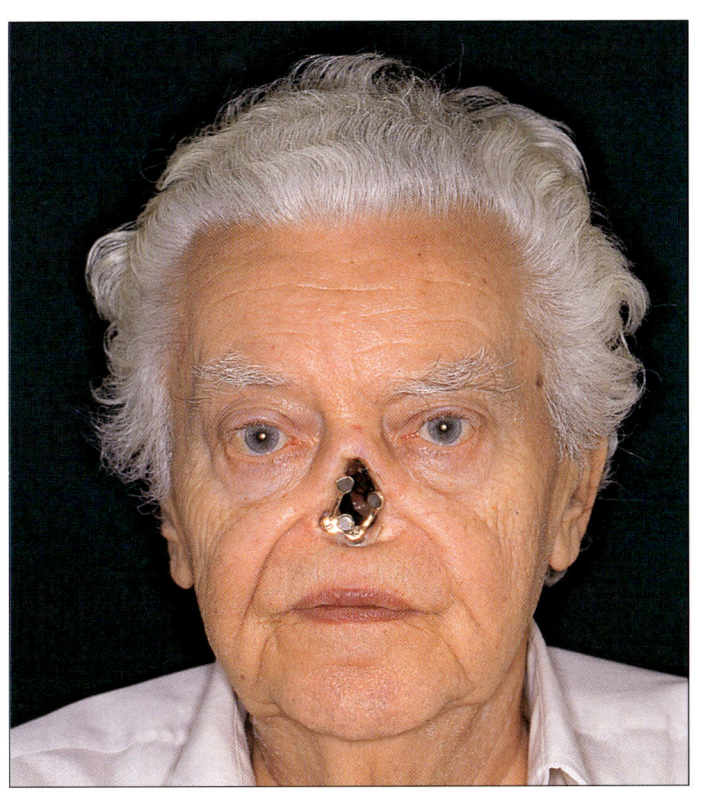
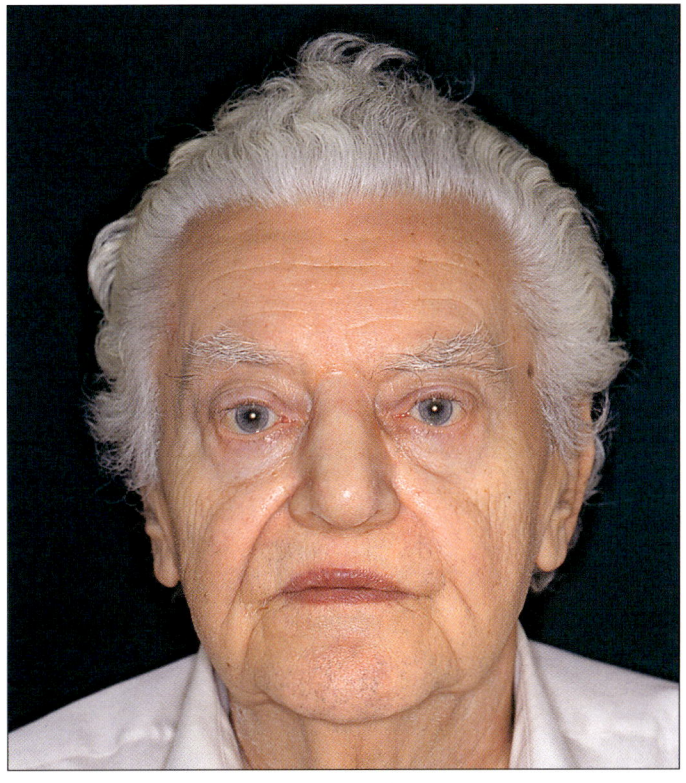
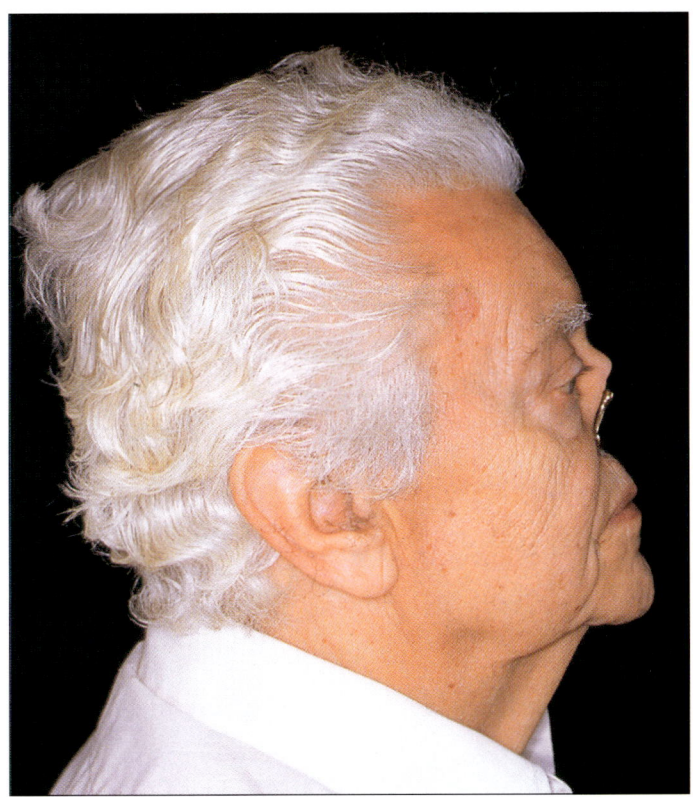
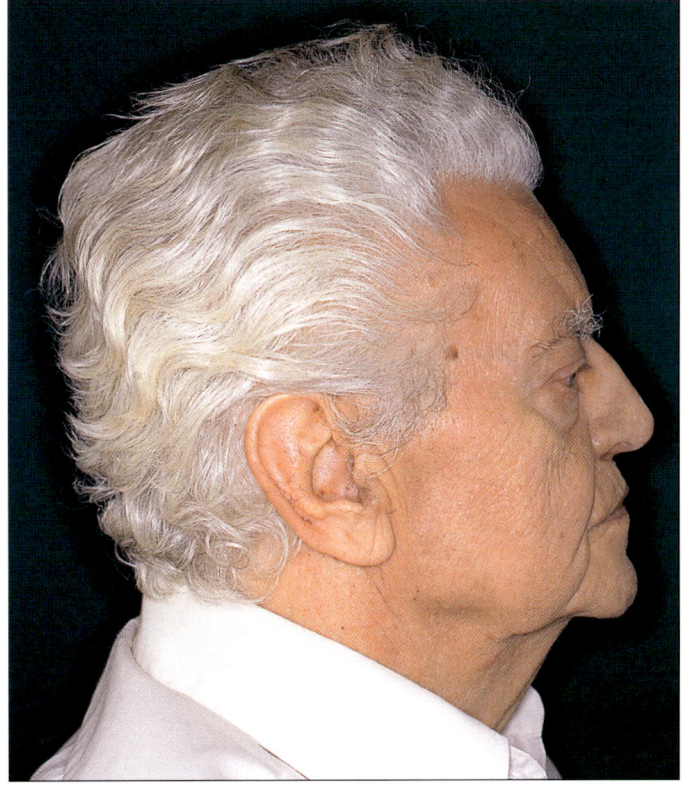

PATIENT PRESENTATION 9

9 This 75-year-old woman underwent a rhinectomy due to basal cell carcinoma in 1985. She was not considered a candidate for nasal reconstruction because of sun damage to her surrounding facial skin. In 1987, three fixtures were placed into the nasal remnant and maxilla, which also involved the extraction of the two central incisor teeth to make room for the fixtures. At second-stage surgery, abutments were connected onto the fixtures. A gold bar was attached to the abutments, and gold clip retention was used on the acrylic base of the silicone nasal prosthesis. (DM)

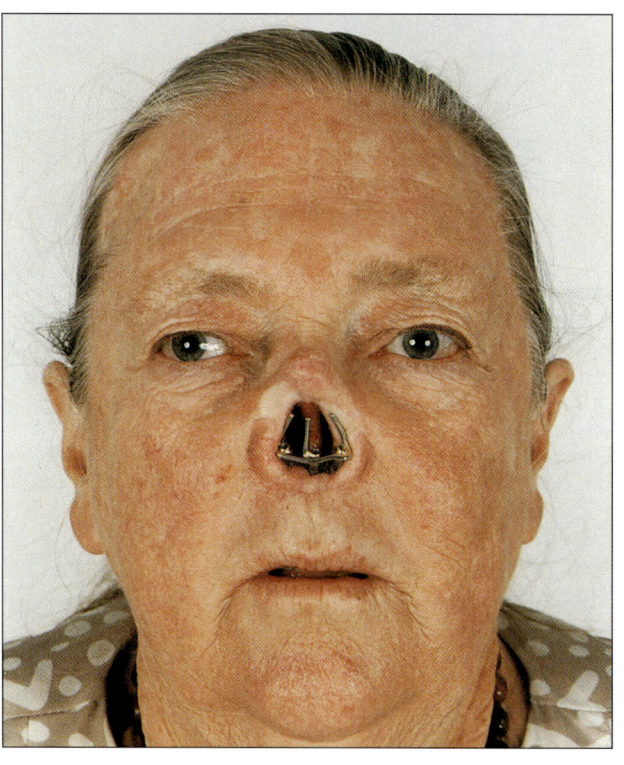

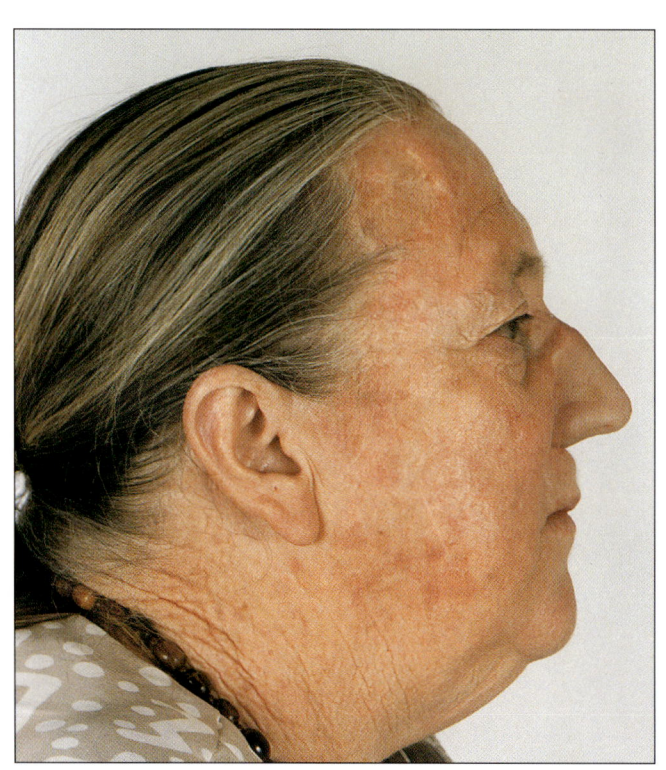

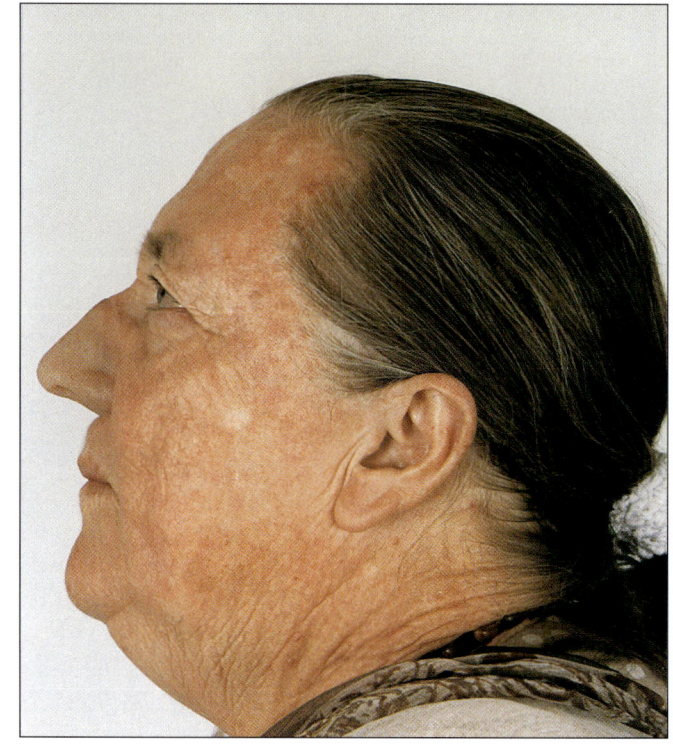

ORBITAL DEFECTS

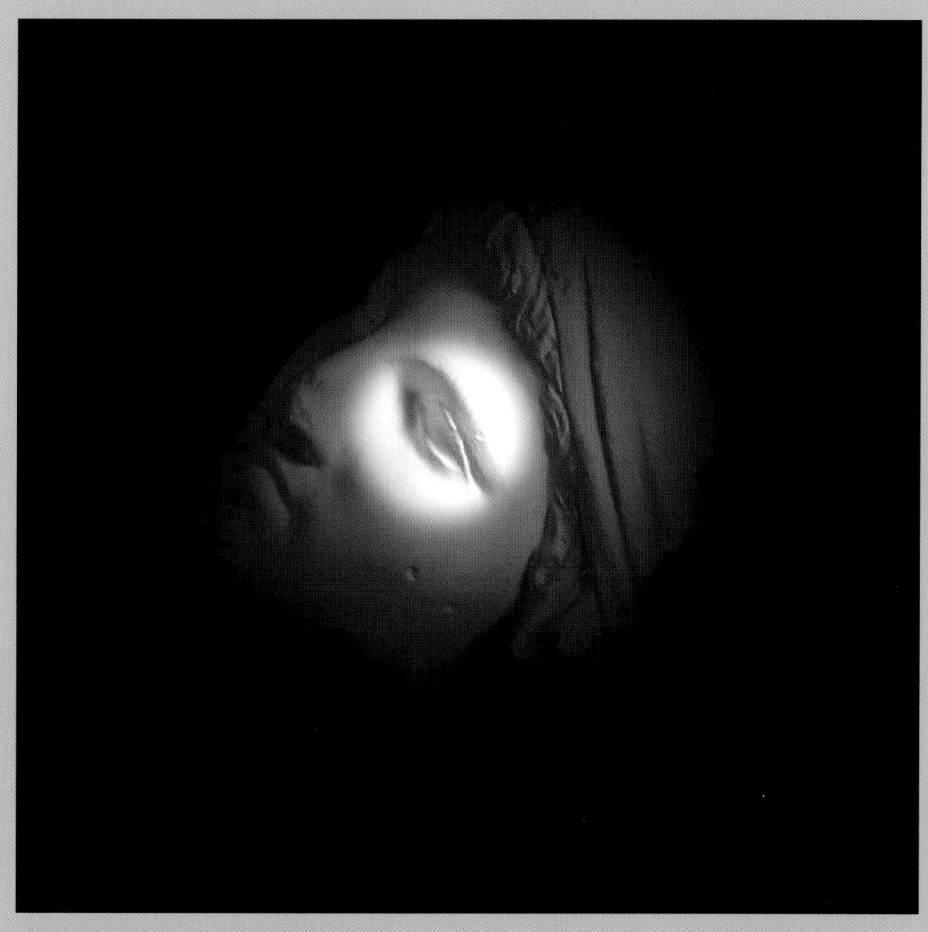

PATIENT PRESENTATION 1

1 This 71-year-old man underwent a left orbital exenteration due to adenocarcinoma of the lacrimal gland. At the same time the tumor was removed, four fixtures were placed in the orbital rim. As part of the treatment plan, he received 62 Gy of radiation postoperatively. Hyperbaric oxygen treatment was not provided because of a heart condition. The orbital prosthesis was retained by individual magnets placed onto the abutments. (KB)

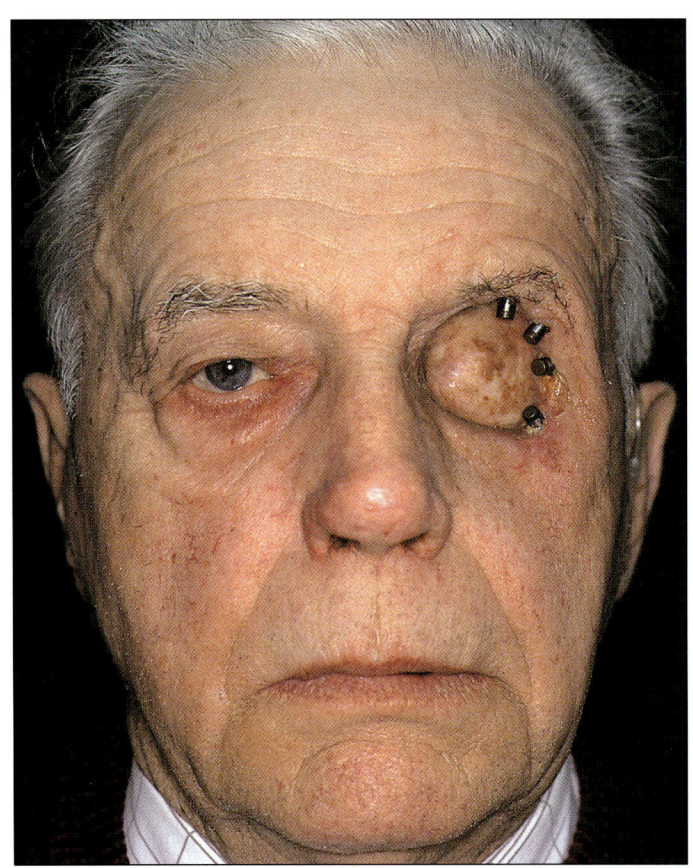
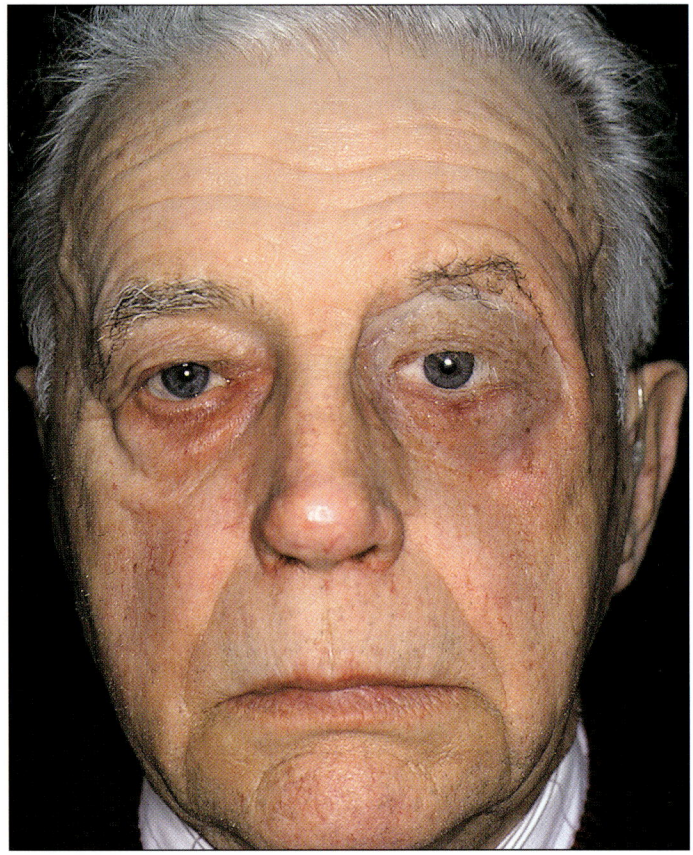
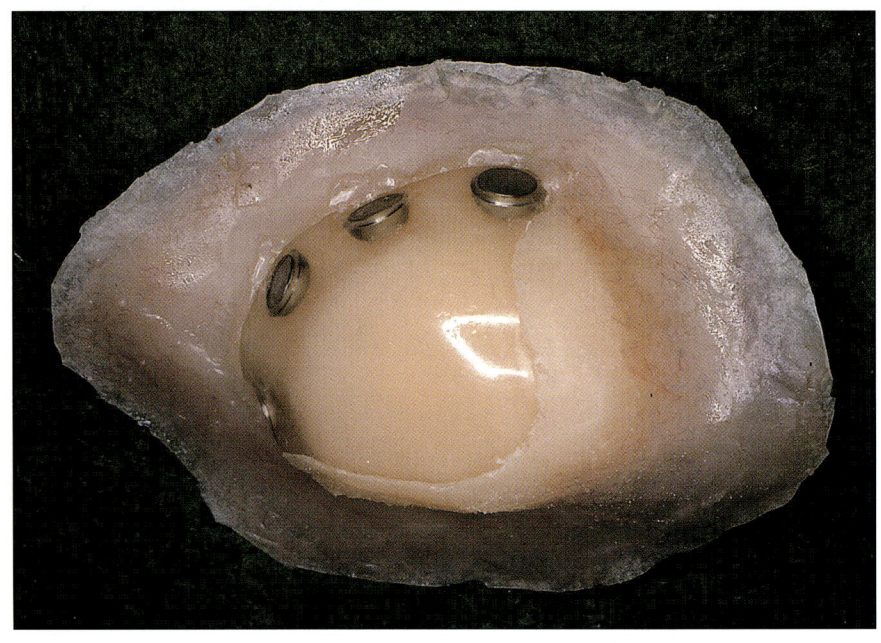

PATIENT PRESENTATION 1

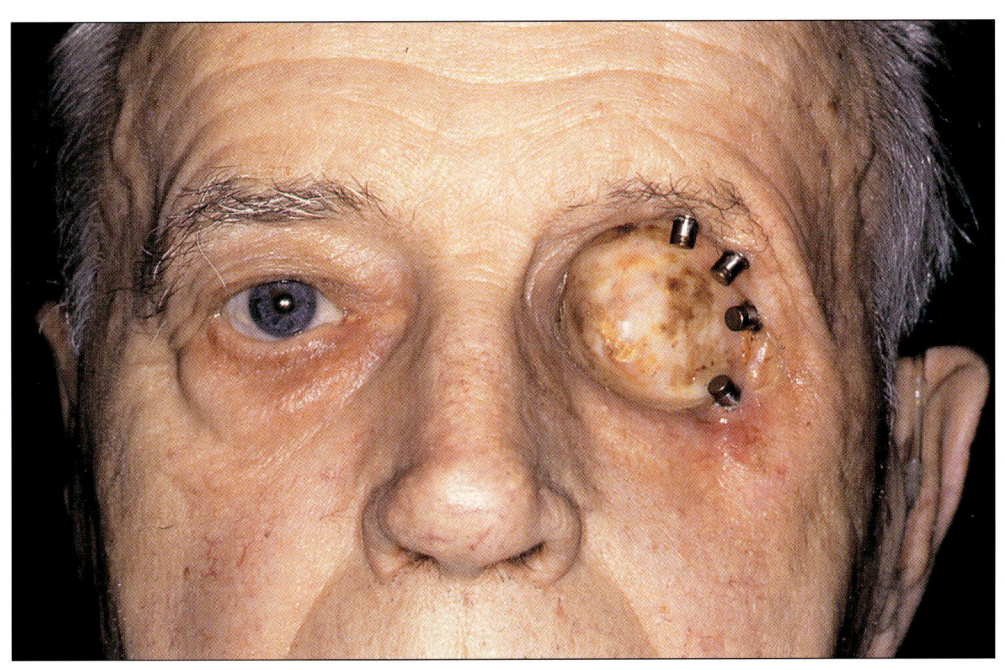

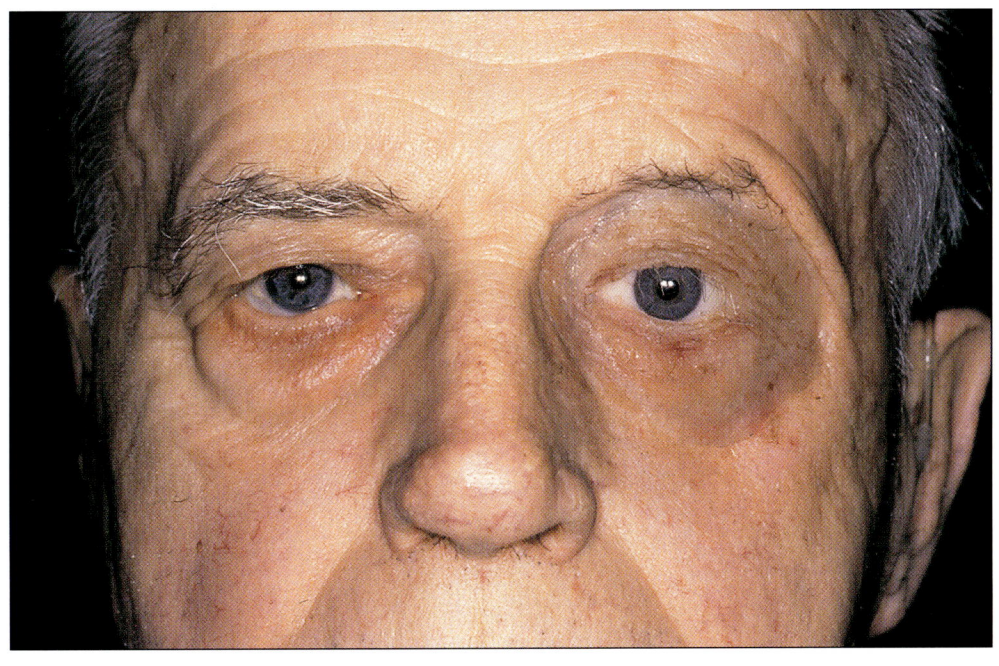

Patient Presentation 2

2 *This 67-year-old man underwent a left orbital exenteration with partial maxillectomy and ethmoidectomy for removal of recurrent basal cell carcinoma of the left orbit and ethmoid complex. A self-retained silicone and acrylic orbital prosthesis was fabricated using the anatomic undercuts for retention. (JB)*

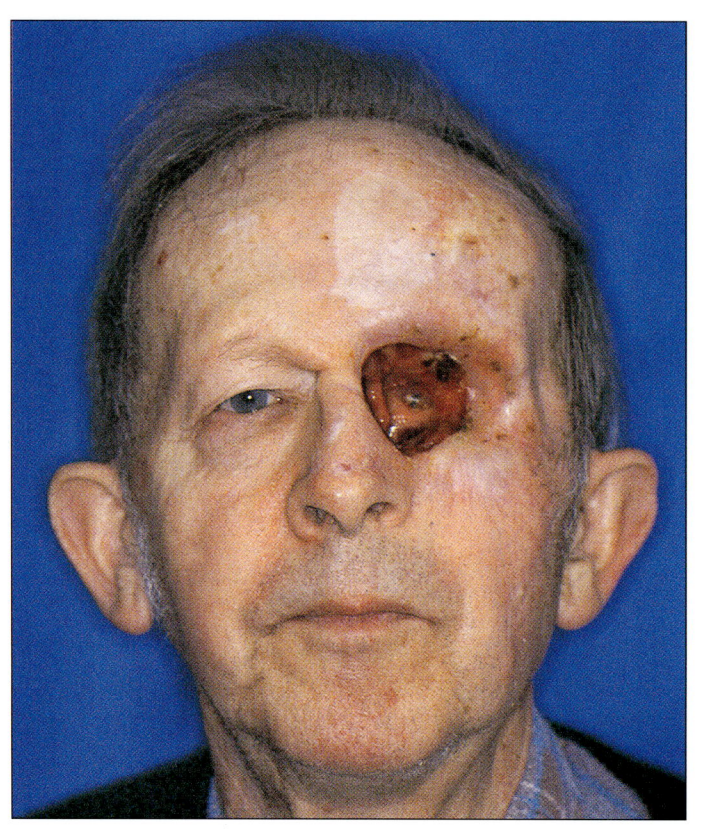
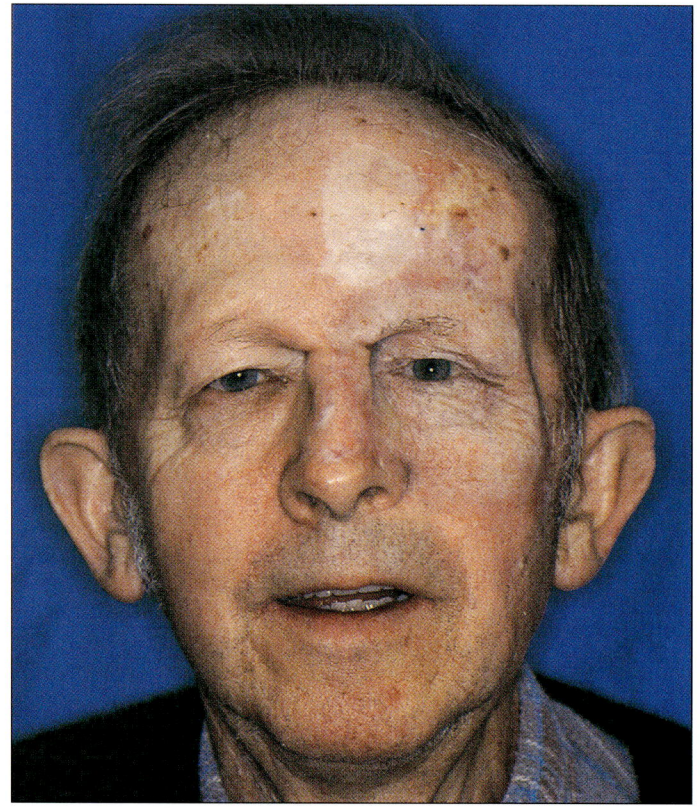
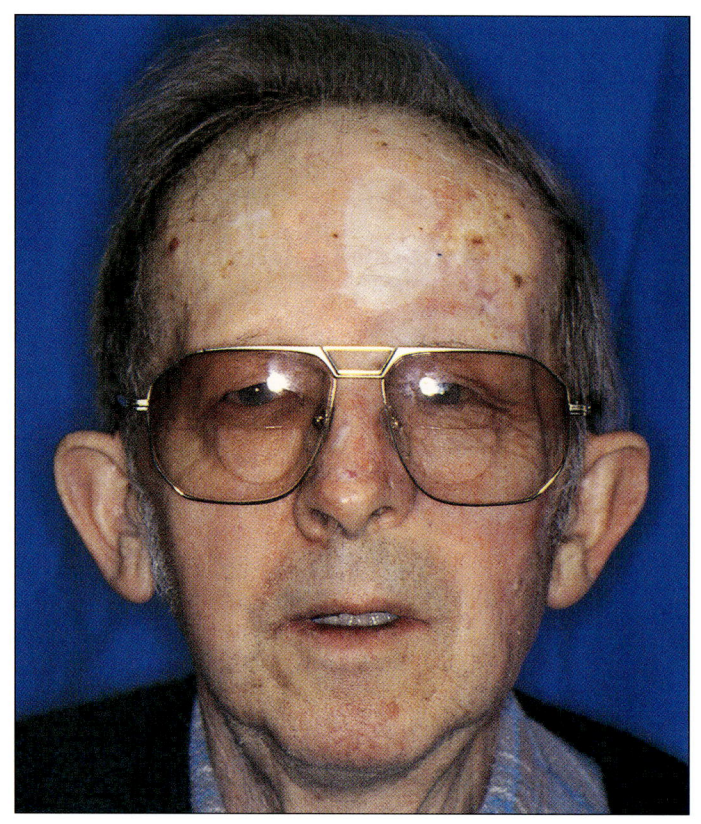

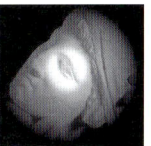

3 This 68-year-old woman underwent a right orbital exenteration due to squamous cell carcinoma. In this particular case, she received an orbital prosthesis retained by medical adhesive. (GD)

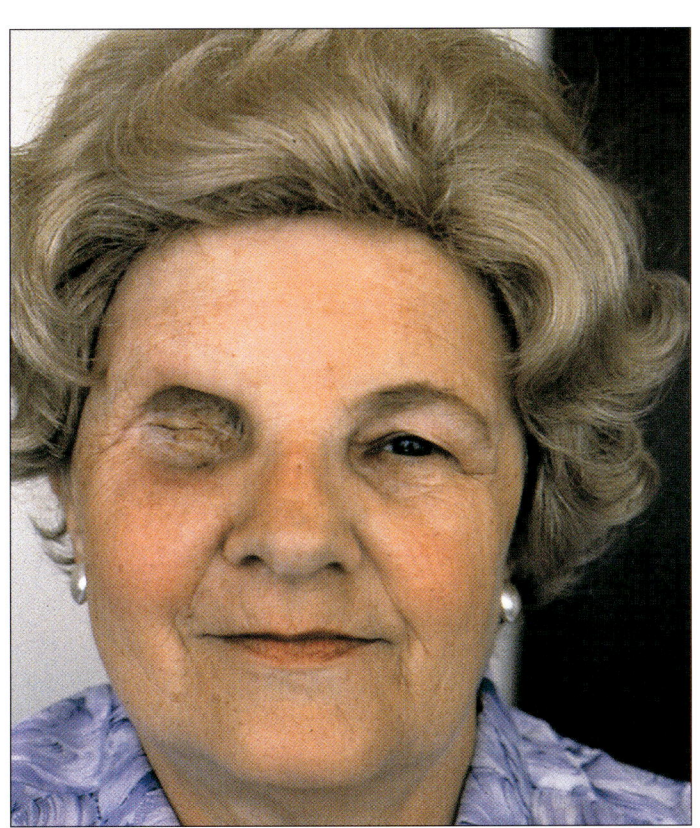
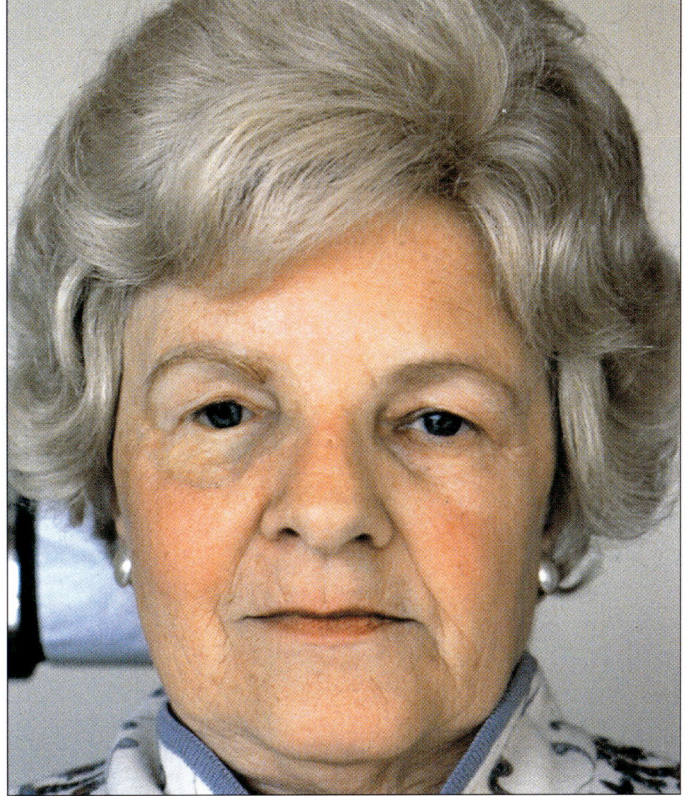
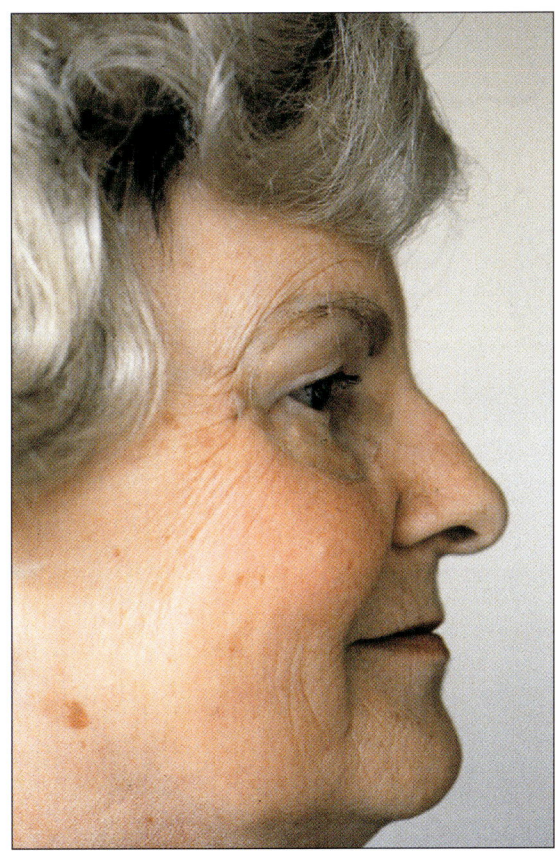

PATIENT PRESENTATION 4

4 This woman underwent a right orbital exenteration due to a rhabdomyosarcoma at the age of 15. In ensuing years, she was fitted with several facial prostheses retained by glasses and adhesives, but none was satisfactory esthetically and functionally since they never felt secure. Eventually, three fixtures were placed in the orbital rim, providing mechanical retention for the prosthesis with a gold bar-and-clip. Later, console abutments were used, providing retention with magnets. (PE)

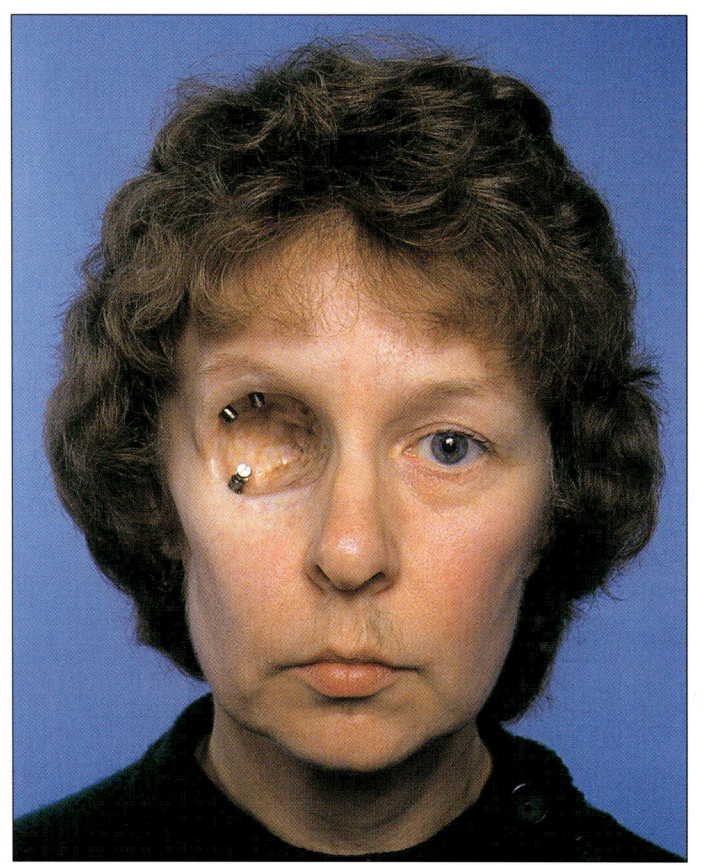
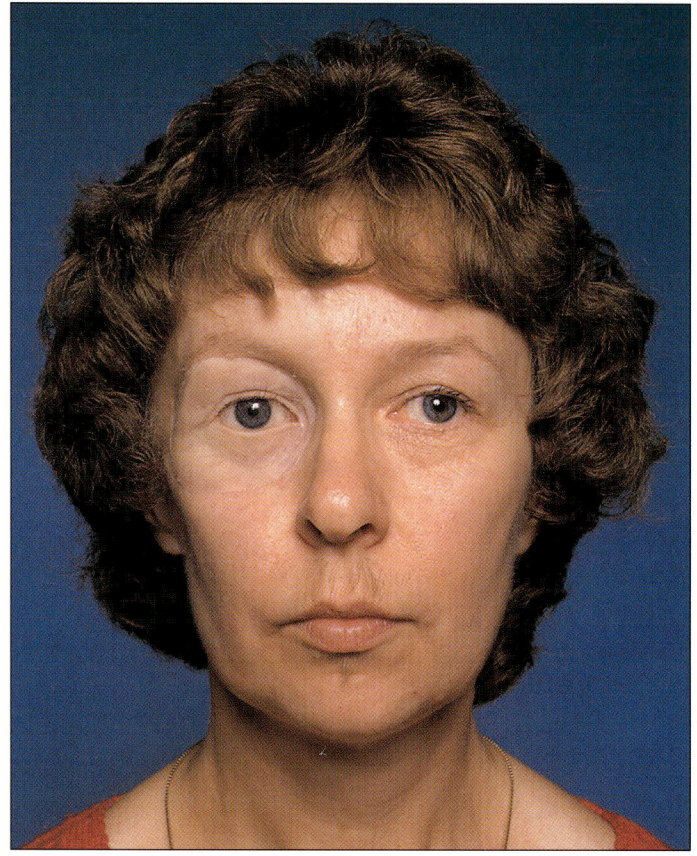
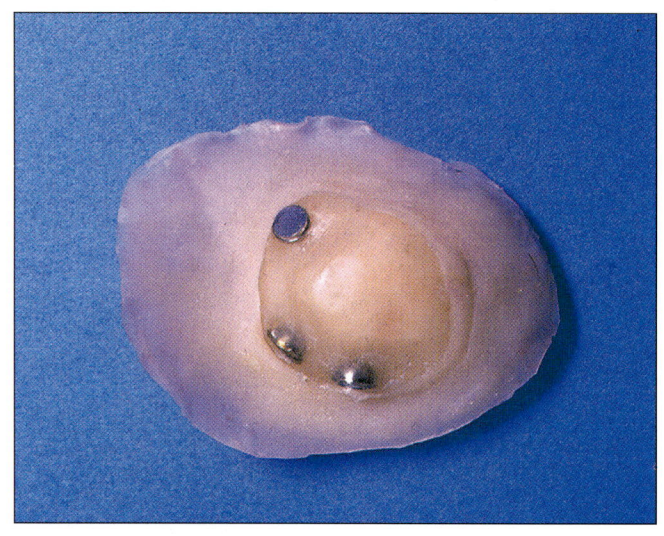

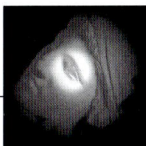

PATIENT PRESENTATION 5

5 *This 67-year-old man underwent a right orbital exenteration due to basal cell carcinoma. He did not receive radiation therapy or chemotherapy. Later on, three fixtures were placed in the orbital rim, and after the healing period, a gold bar with two magnets was fabricated, providing retention for the prosthesis. (AF)*

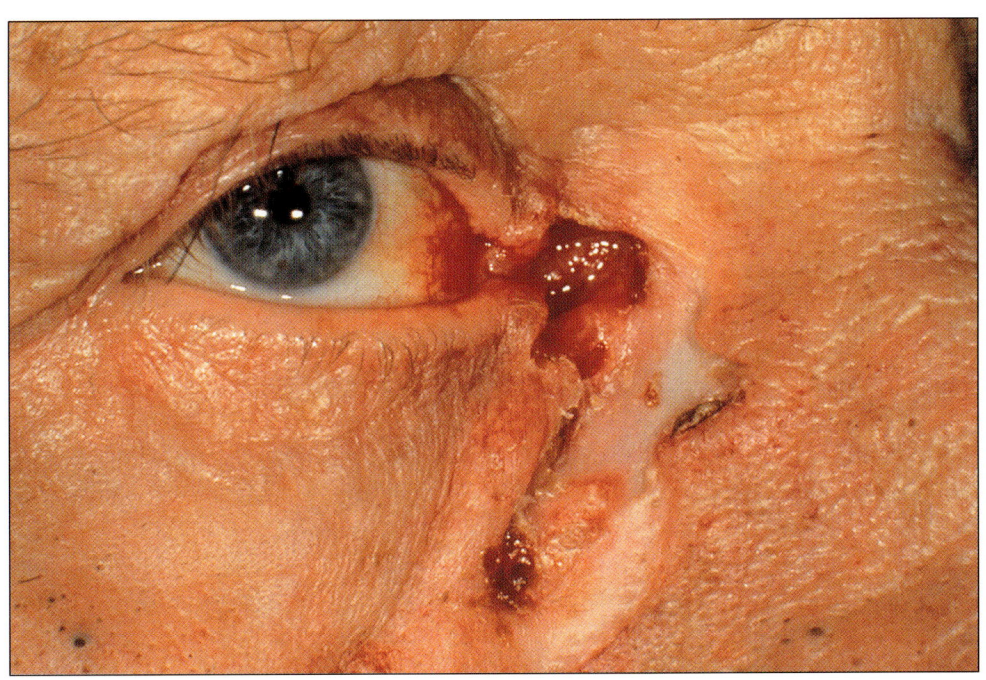

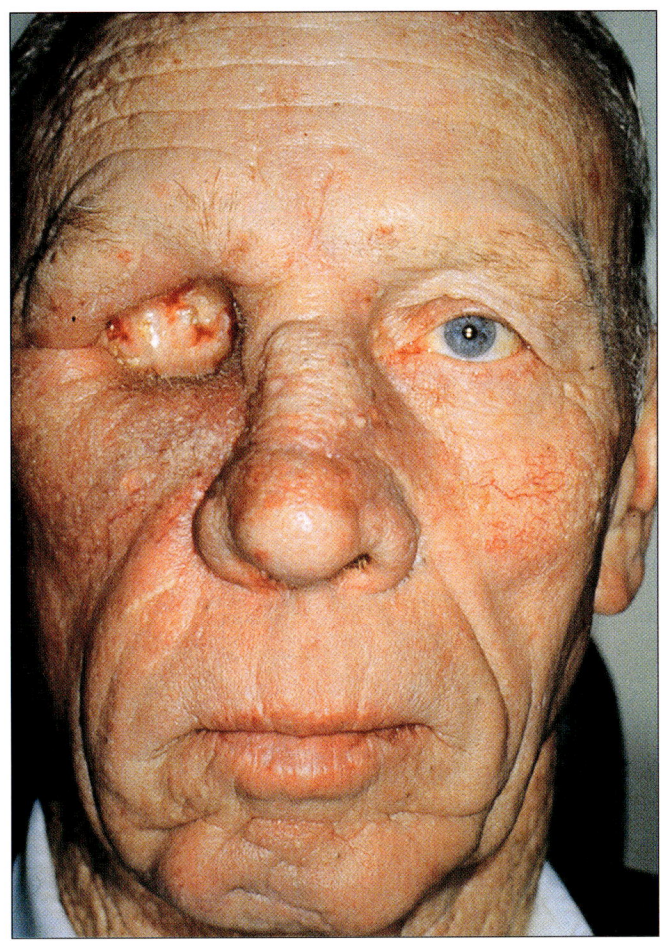

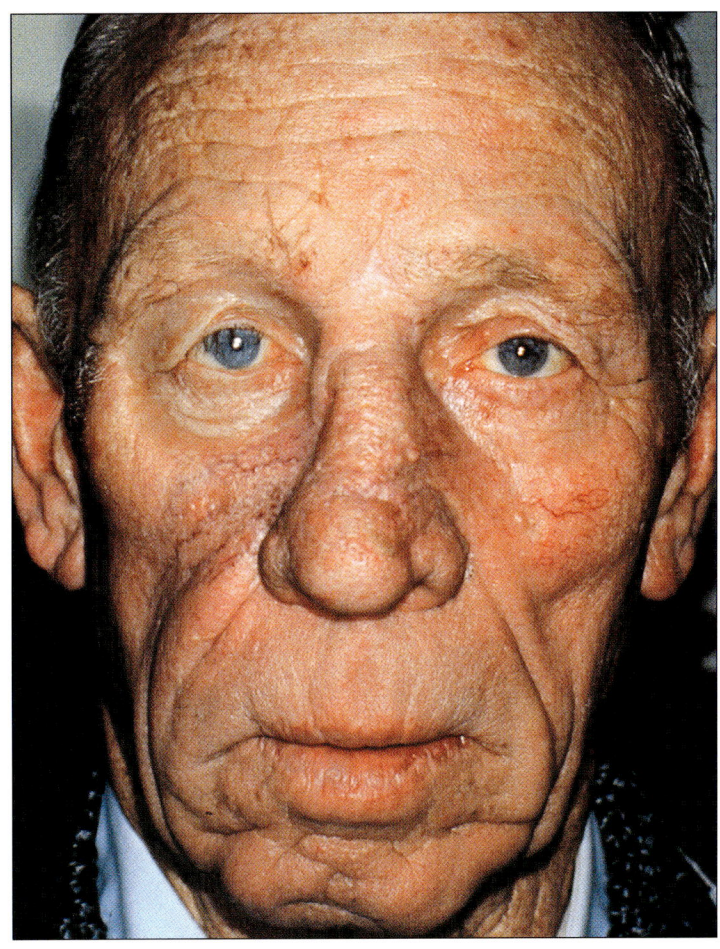

(continued)

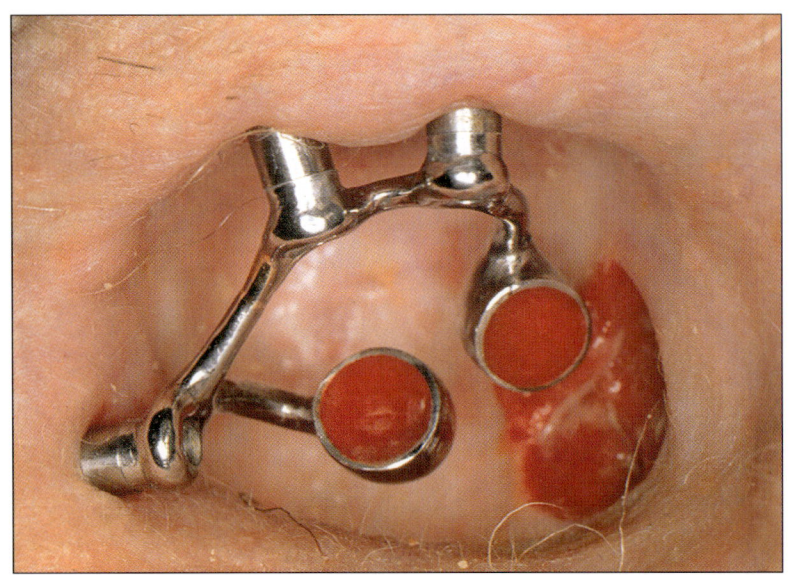
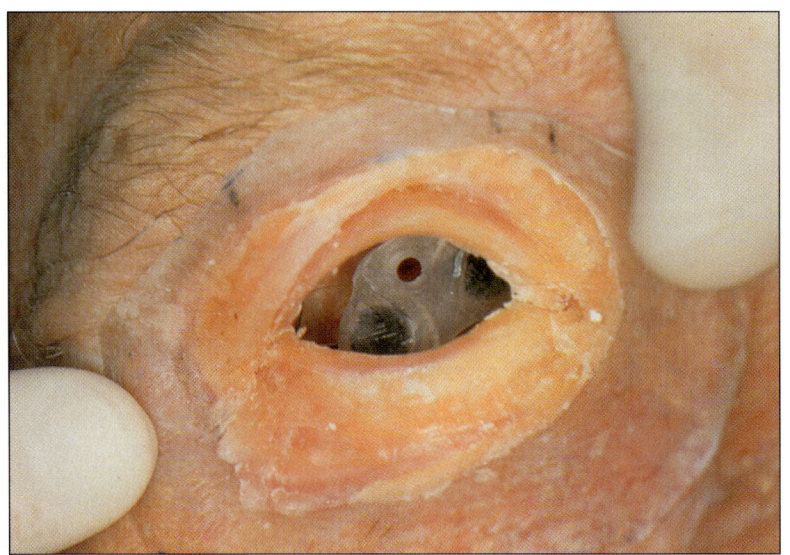
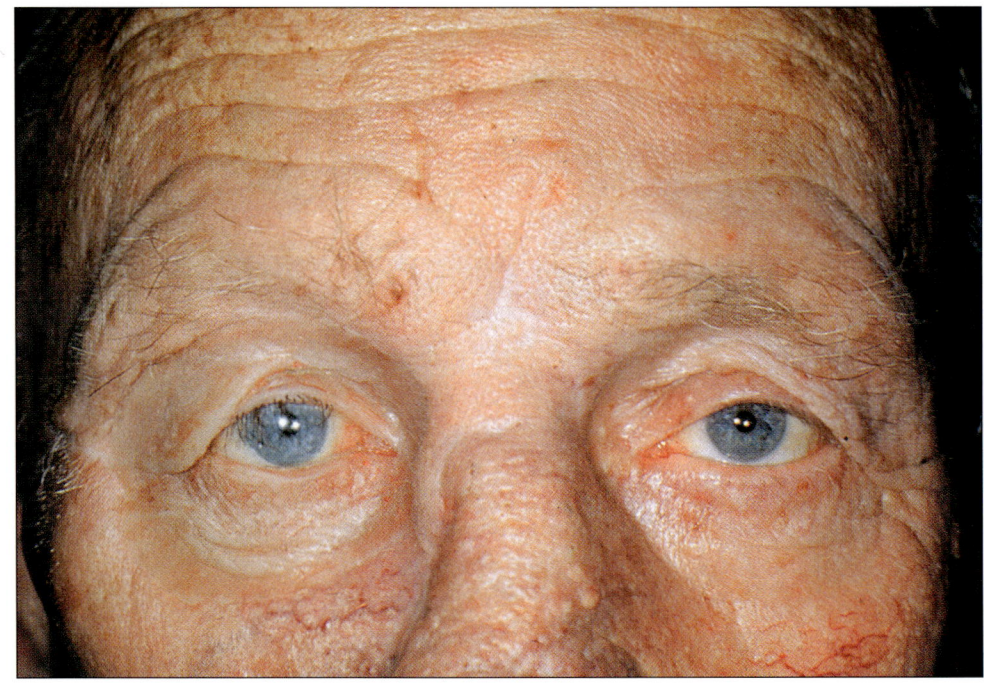

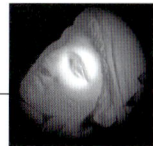

PATIENT PRESENTATION 6

6 *This 71-year-old woman underwent a right orbital exenteration due to meibomian gland carcinoma. When the soft tissue healed, an adhesive-retained silicone orbital prosthesis was fitted, restoring the missing facial structure. (AF)*

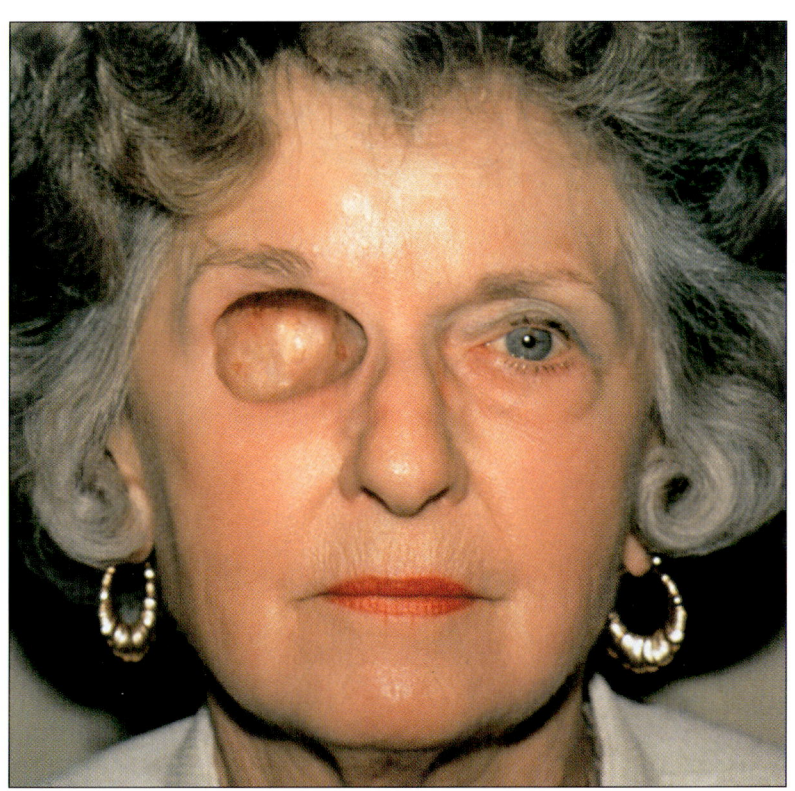

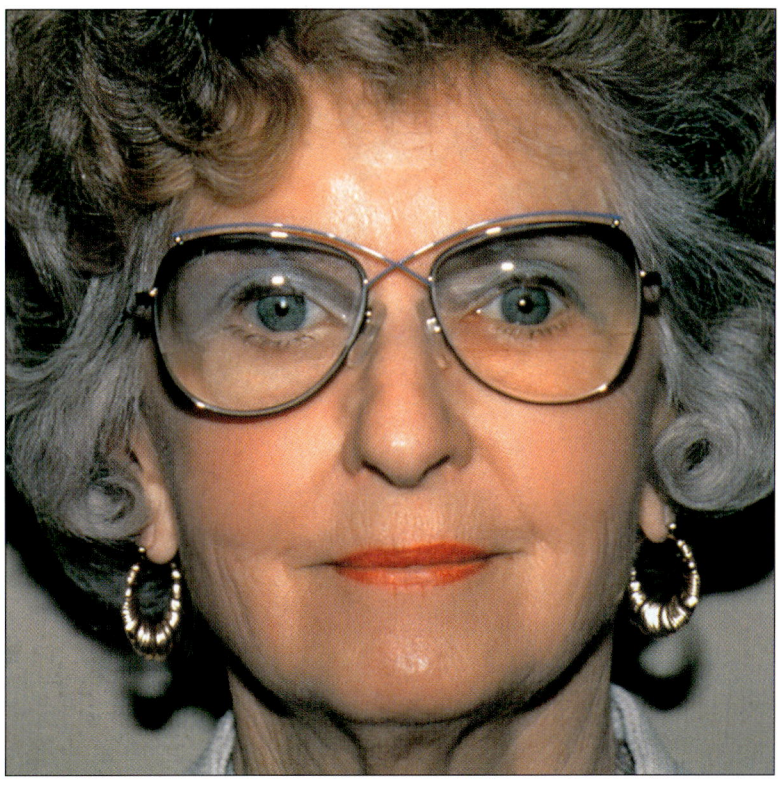

7

This 58-year-old woman underwent a left orbital exenteration due to a meningioma. After the healing period, she was provided with an anatomically retained, hollow bulb orbital prosthesis. (GG)

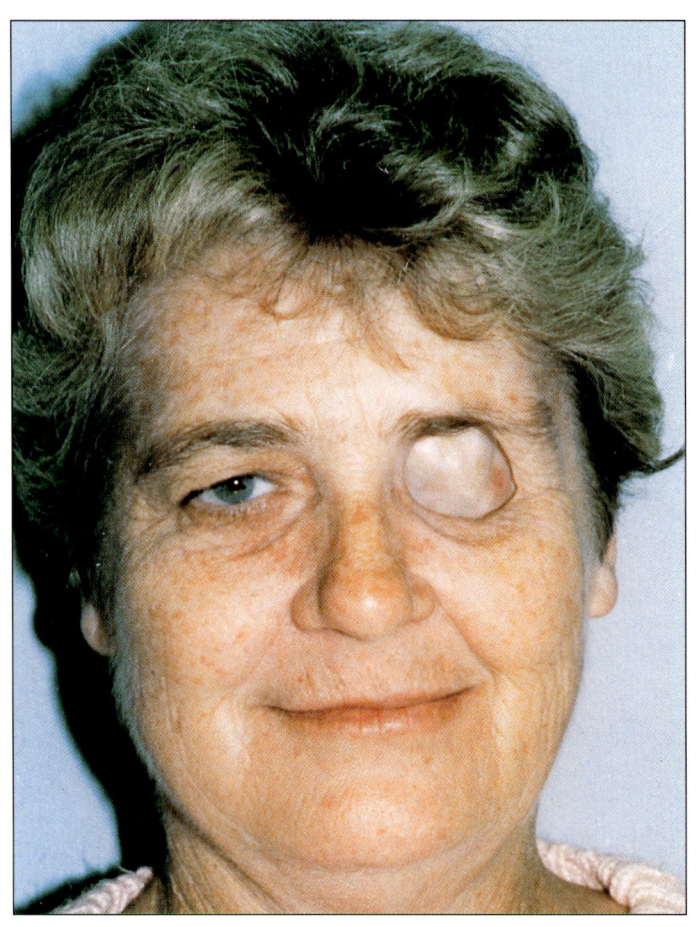
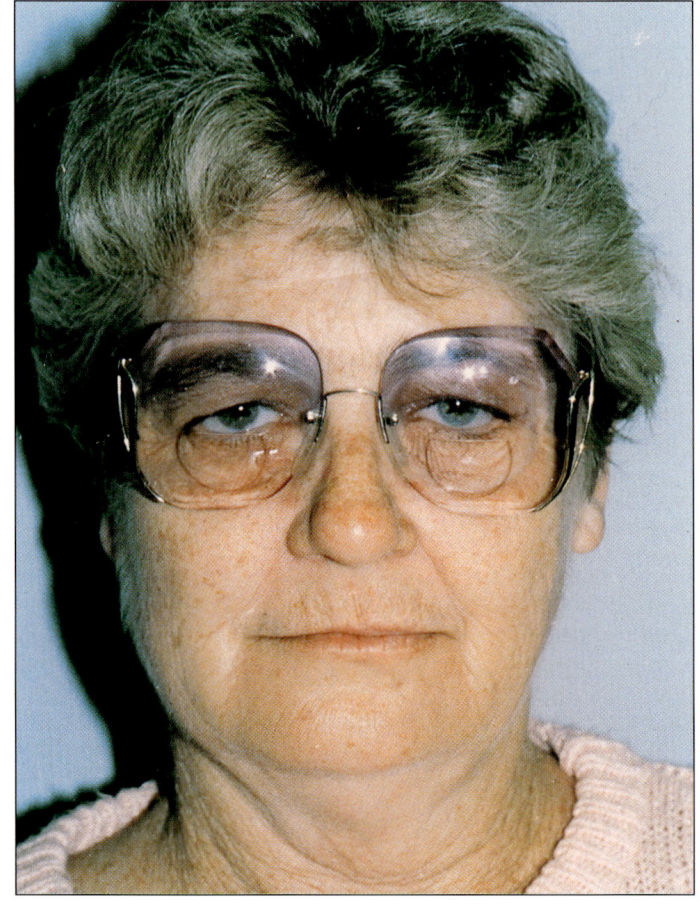
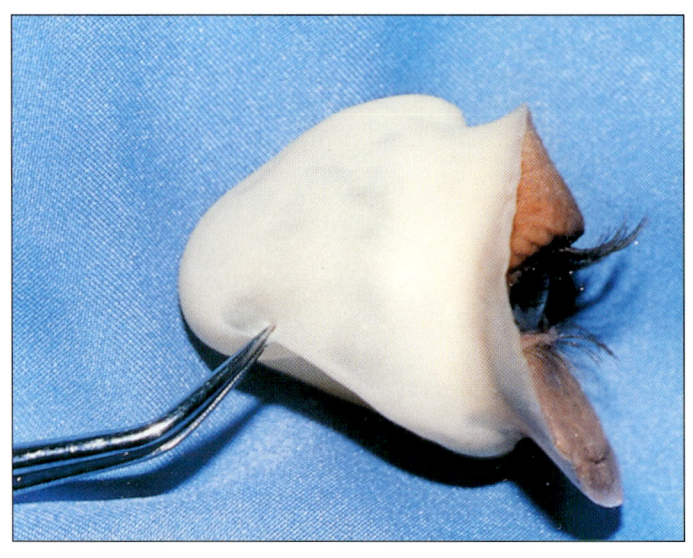
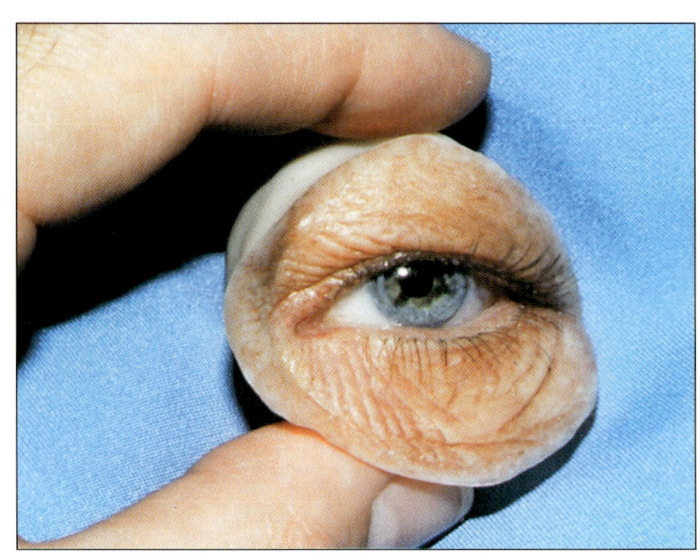

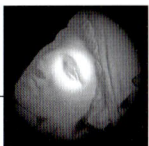

8 *This 74-year-old woman underwent a right orbital exenteration due to squamous cell carcinoma of the skin that invaded the orbit and ethmoid sinus. She was provided with a silicone orbital prosthesis, retained by a combination of adhesive and anatomic undercuts. (GG)*

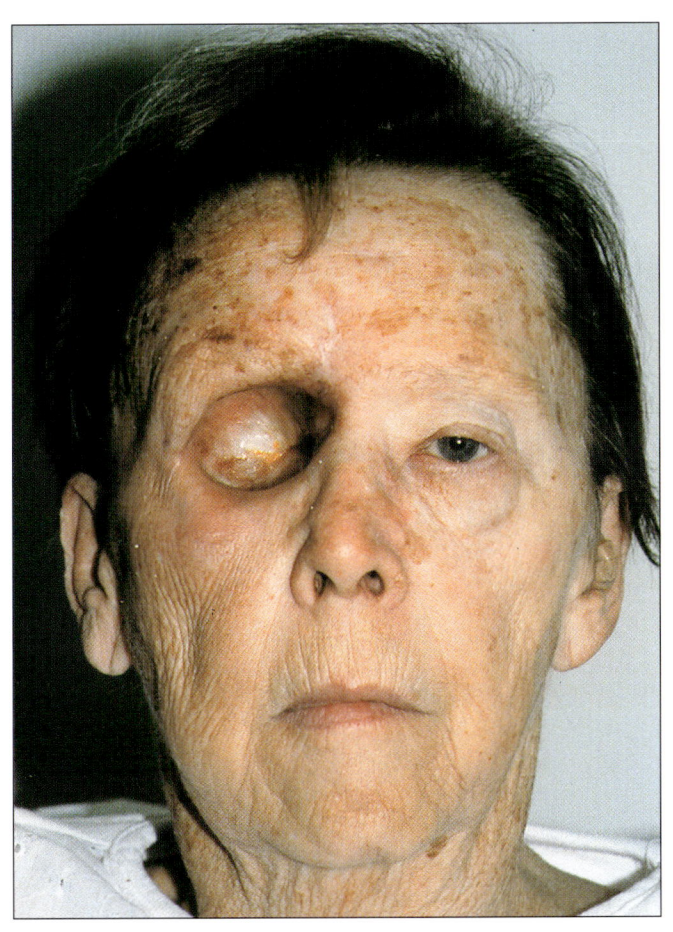
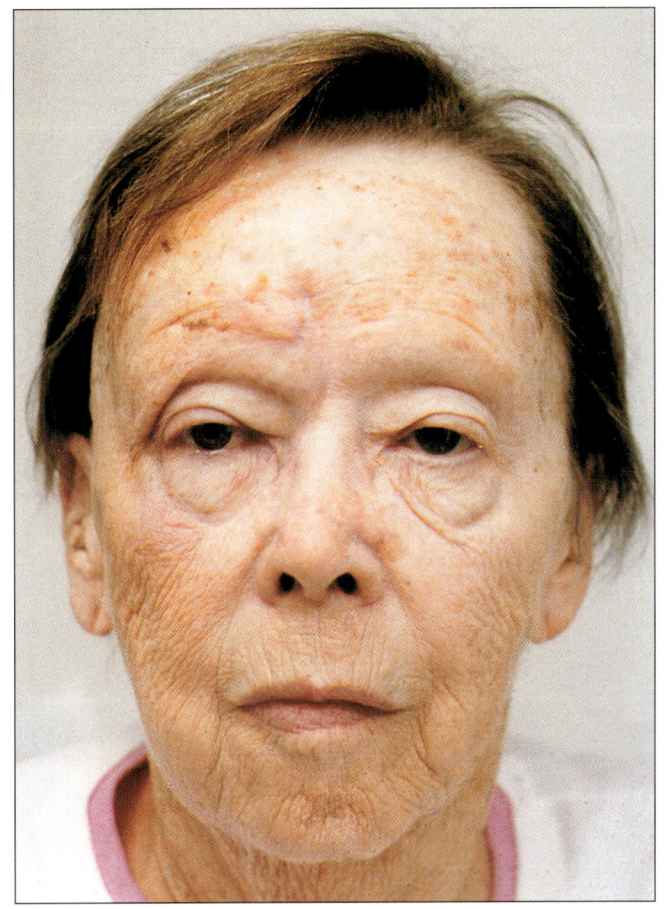
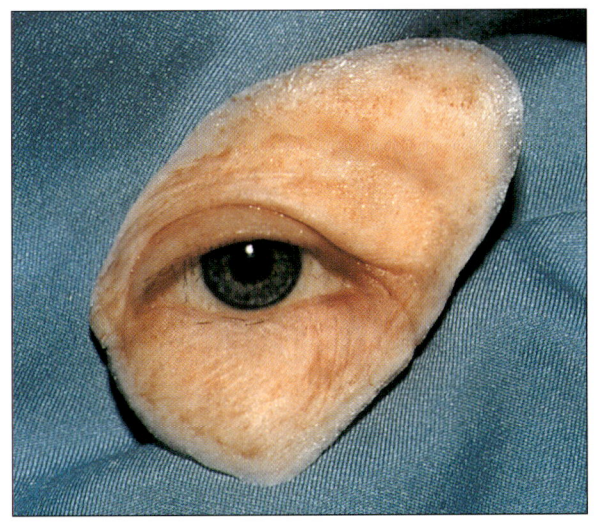

Patient Presentation 9

9 *This 69-year-old woman underwent a right orbital exenteration due to malignant melanoma. After the healing period, an adhesive-retained silicone prosthesis was fabricated for the patient. (PS)*

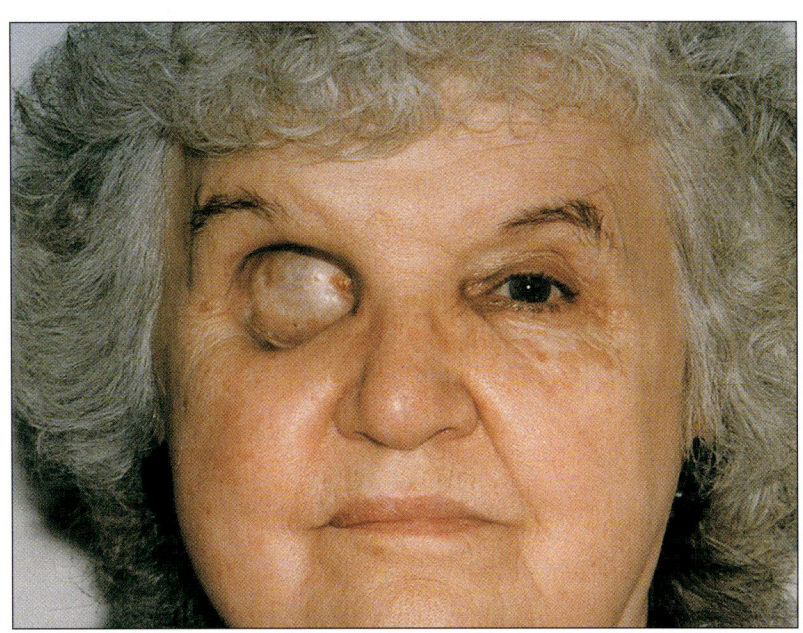

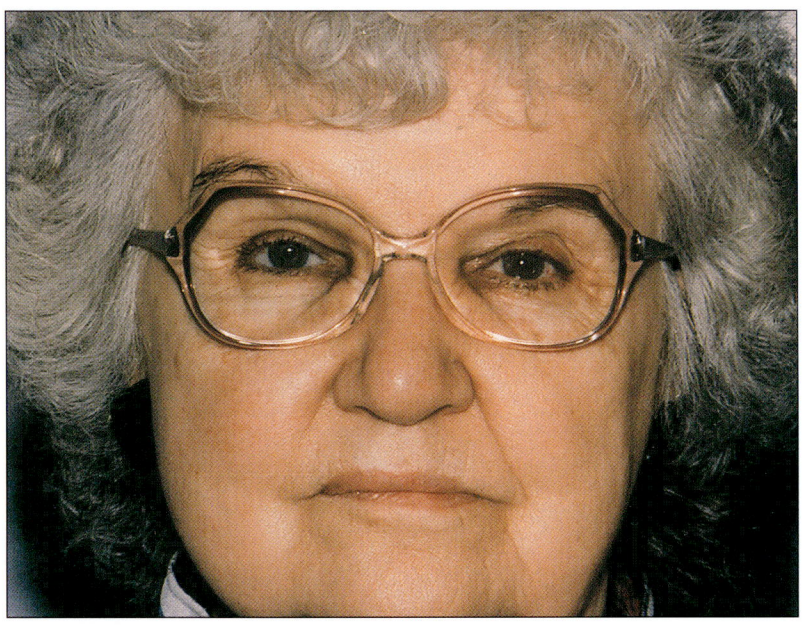

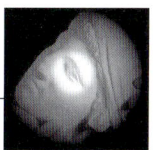

Patient Presentation 10

10 This 64-year-old woman underwent an excision of the right lower eyelid. Residual tumor eventually invaded the orbit, for which a complete exenteration was performed. Options regarding the retention of the prosthesis were given to the patient, who decided to have osseointegrated anchorage. Since it was planned as a single-stage procedure, three fixtures were placed in the orbital rim, and three 4.0-mm abutments were connected to them. Three months after surgery, an impression was made to begin fabrication of the prosthesis. Because of the size of the defect, position of fixtures, patient manual dexterity, and lack of displaced soft-tissue movement, magnetic retention was the method of choice. The prosthesis was then fabricated and fitted, allowing the patient to return to a normal life. (KT)

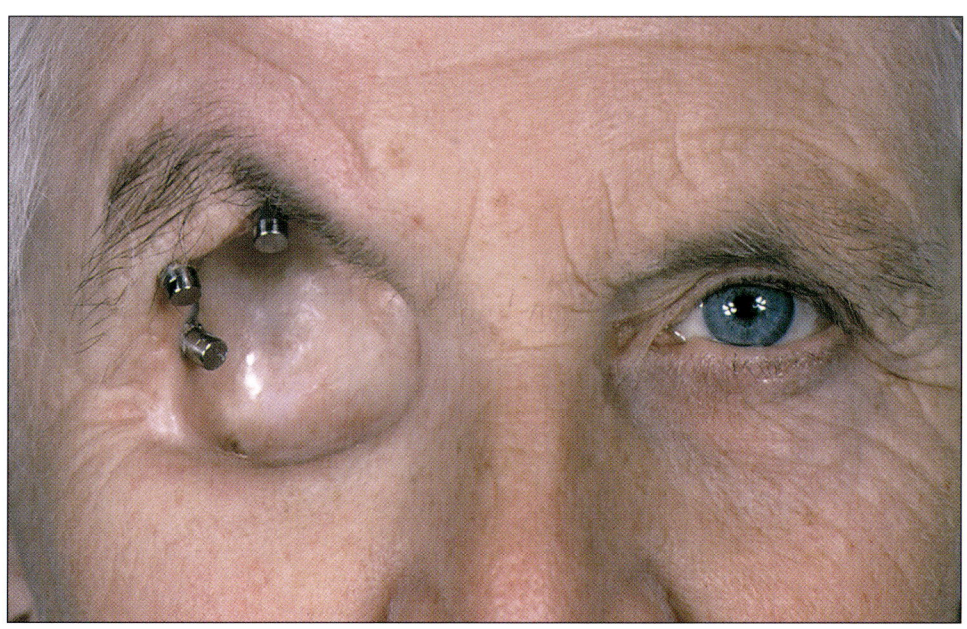

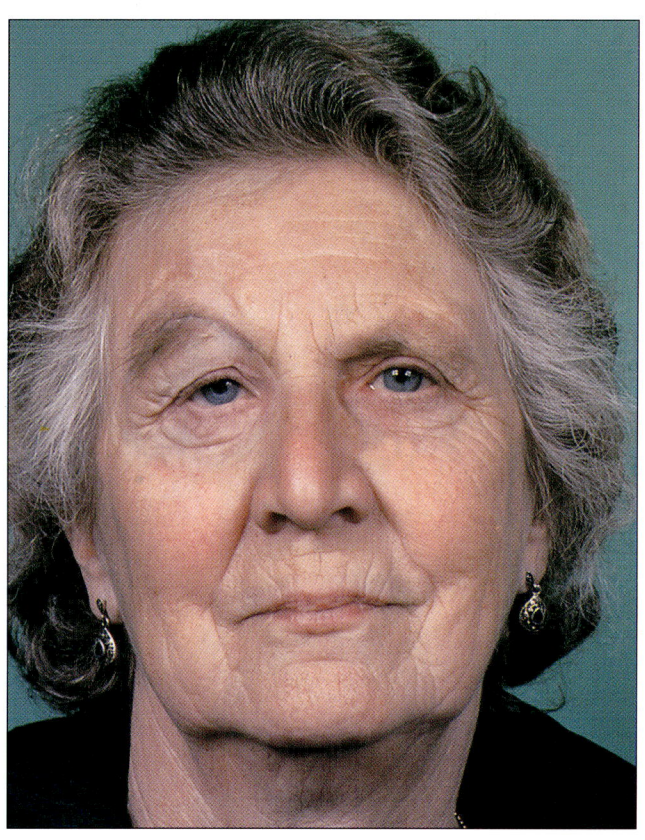

11 *This 82-year-old man underwent a right orbital exenteration due to basal cell carcinoma. He did not receive radiation therapy. After the healing period, four fixtures were placed in the orbital rim to provide retention for a silicone orbital prosthesis.* (DT)

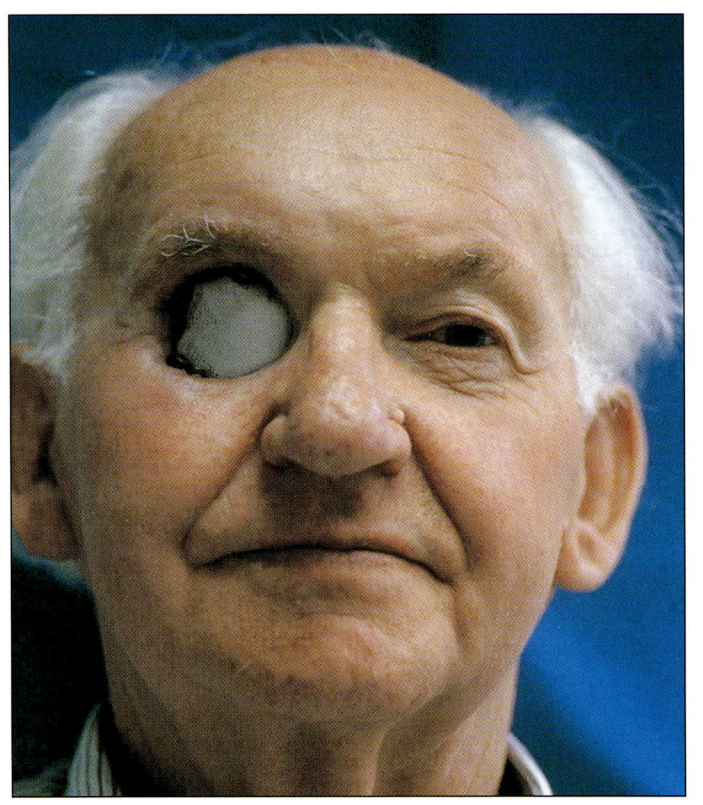
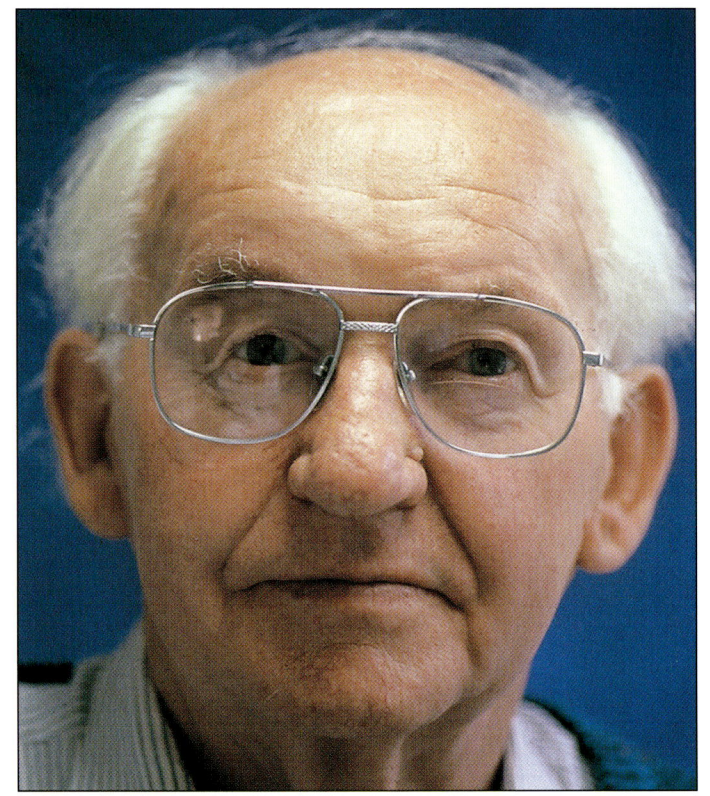

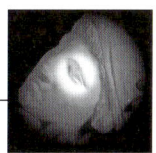

12 This 84-year-old man underwent a left orbital exenteration due to a carcinoma of the left eyelid. He did not receive radiation therapy. After the placement of three osseointegrated fixtures, an orbital silicone prosthesis was retained by three magnets connected to the abutments. (DT)

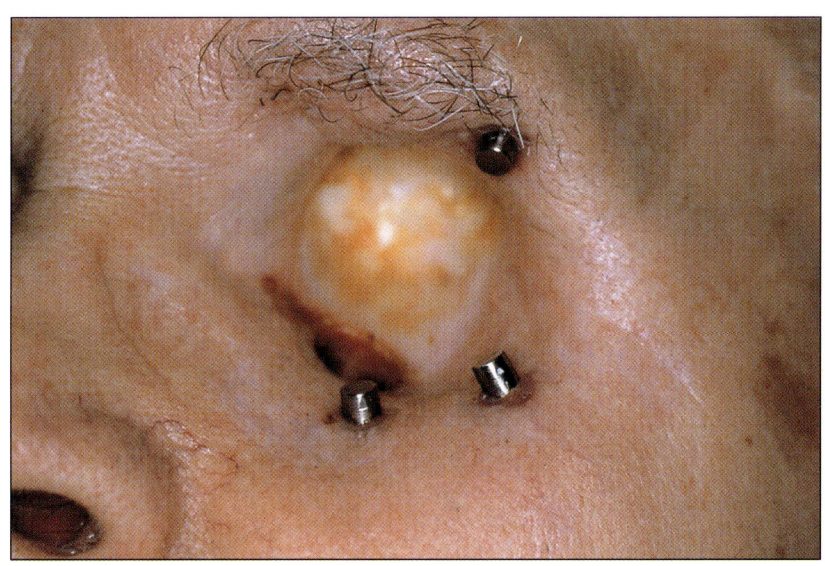

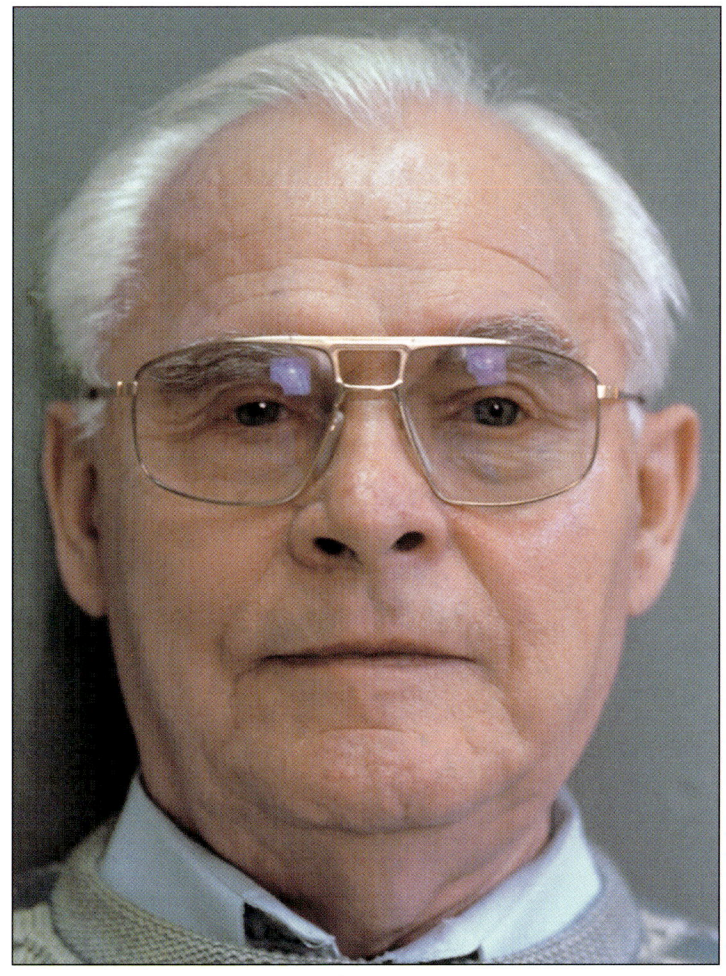

13 This 59-year-old woman was first seen at our unit in August 1988 wearing a spectacle-mounted orbital prosthesis for a right traumatically acquired defect from a road traffic accident in 1961. The patient's main concern was the stability of the prosthesis, particularly when caring for her grandchildren. Her situation was considered suitable for an osseointegrated orbital prosthesis; three fixtures were placed in the orbital rim in October 1988. The silicone orbital prosthesis was initially fitted with gold bar and clips. This gave adequate retention, but the patient had difficulty cleaning around the bar, which was replaced with individual magnets. No prosthetic problems were observed until July 1993, when one fixture was removed due to loss of osseointegration. Two additional fixtures were placed, and no further complications have occurred. (SW)

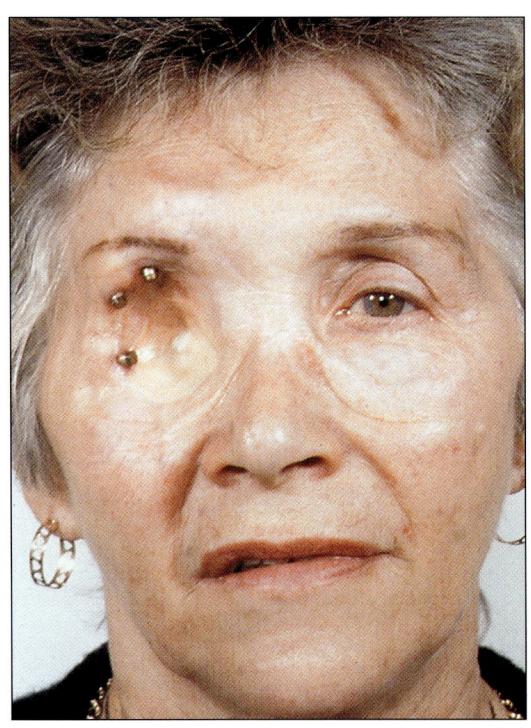
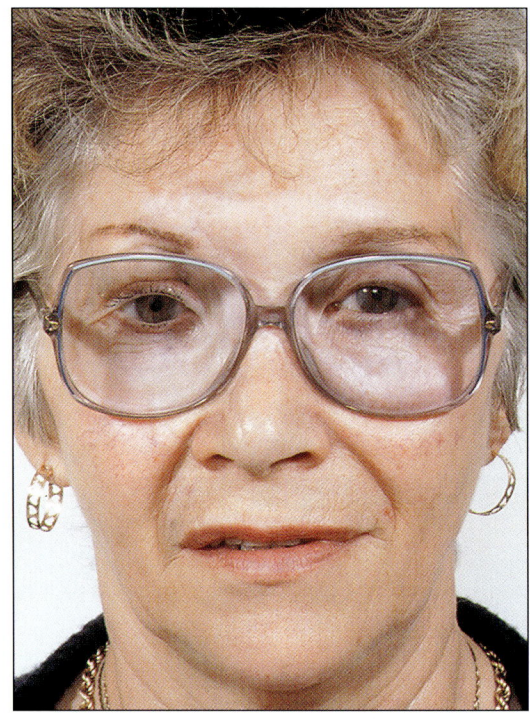
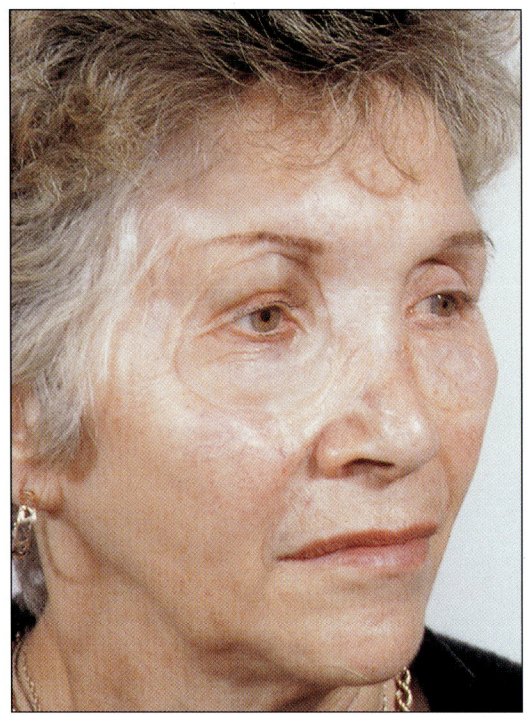

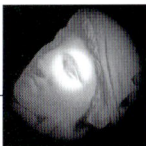

14 *This 71-year-old woman underwent a right orbital exenteration and medial maxillectomy due to squamous cell carcinoma of the lacrimal gland. She also received postoperative radiation therapy at a total dose of 56 Gy. After the healing period, an adhesive-retained silicone prosthesis was fabricated. (LM)*

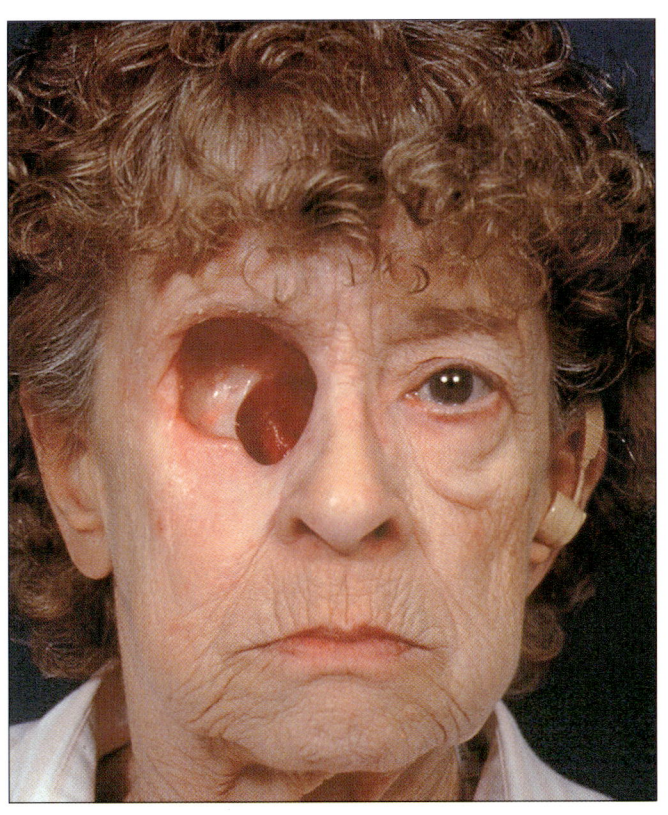
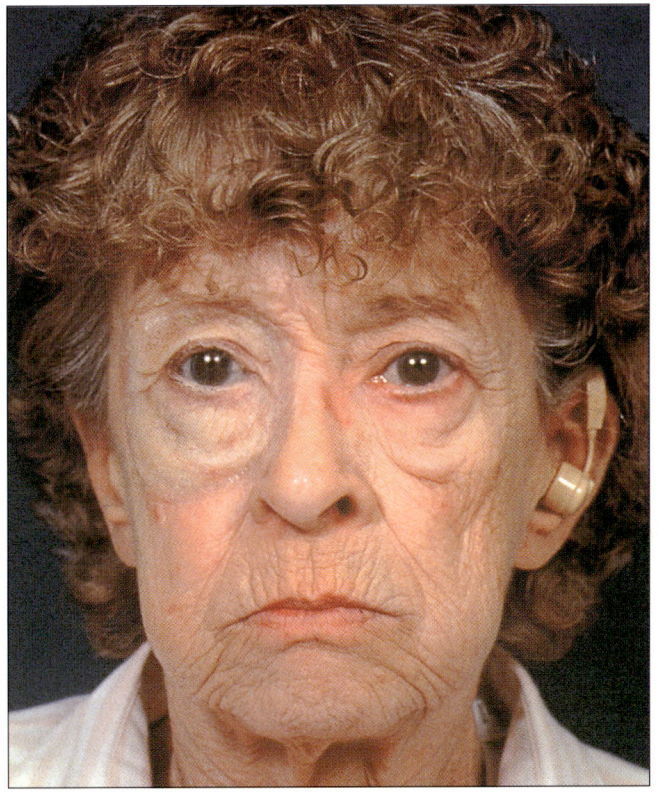
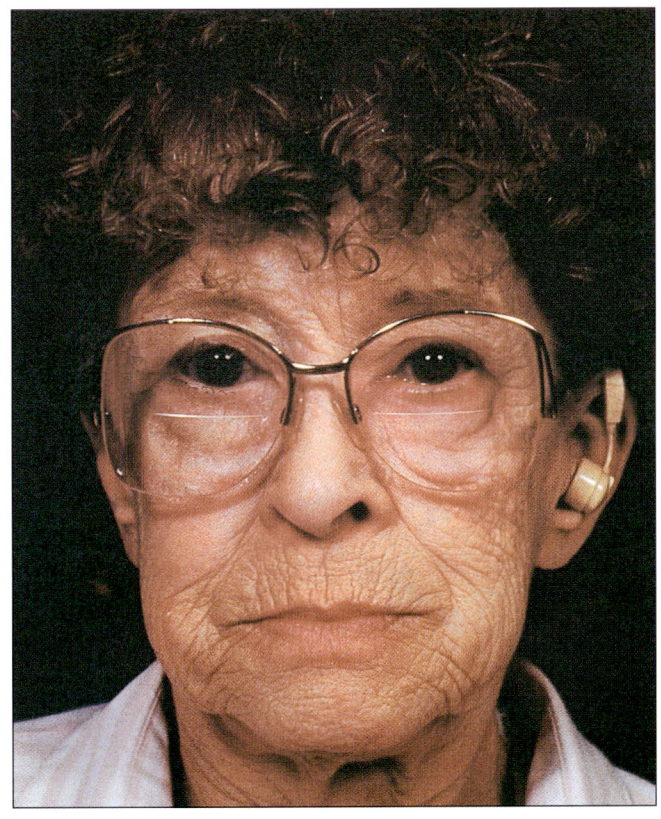

15 This 55-year-old woman underwent a right wide resection of temporal bone and orbital exenteration due to an extensive basal cell carcinoma. During the following year, four osseointegrated implants were placed in the orbital rim in a two-stage procedure, and the patient was fitted with a silicone orbital prosthesis retained by four magnets. (SG)

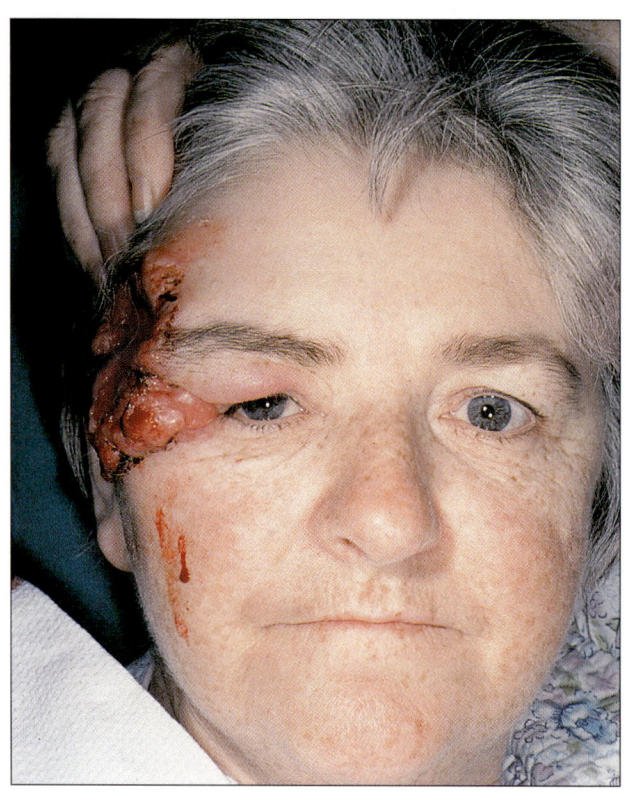
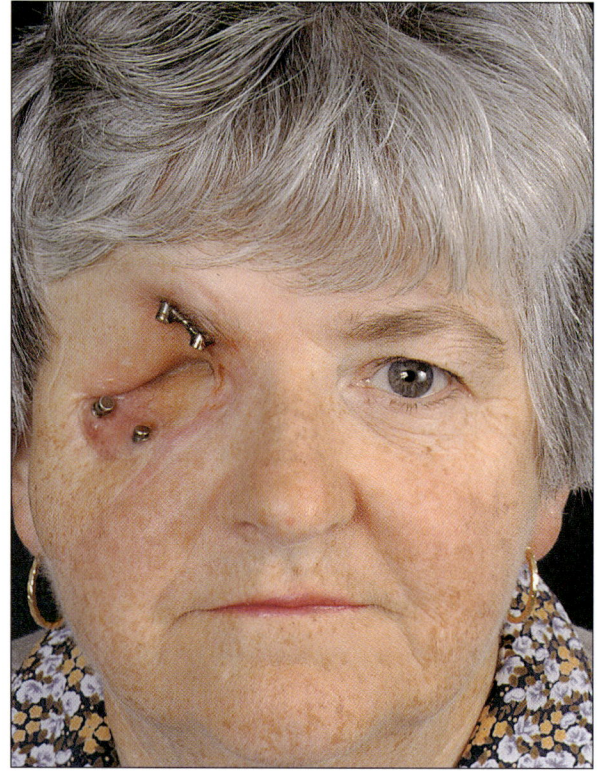
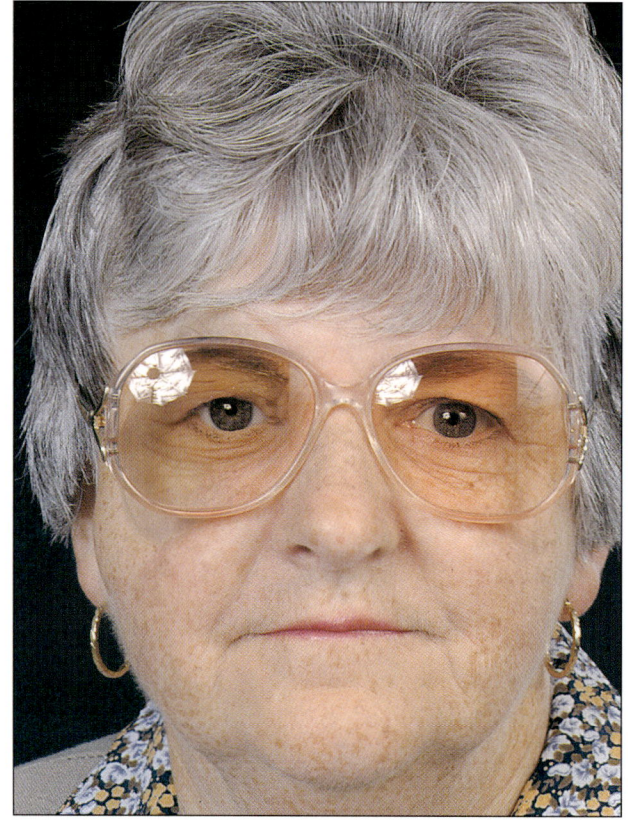

COMPLEX DEFECTS

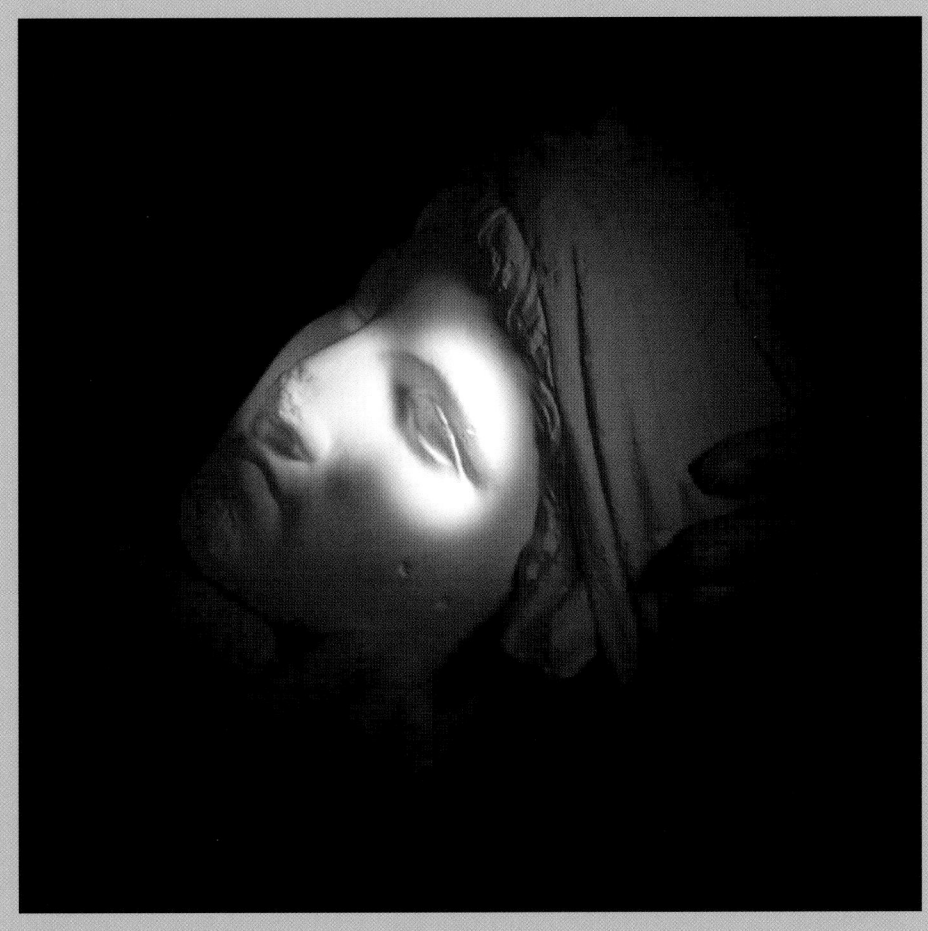

PATIENT PRESENTATION 1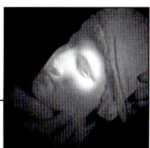

1 *This 51-year-old man suffered a gunshot wound in the submental area. He underwent several surgical procedures, including a bone graft free flap. Later, osseointegrated implants were placed to anchor an obdurator in the upper jaw and a fixed bridge in the lower jaw. The silicone nasal prosthesis was retained by a bar with a clip and magnet, fitted on two fixtures. (LM)*

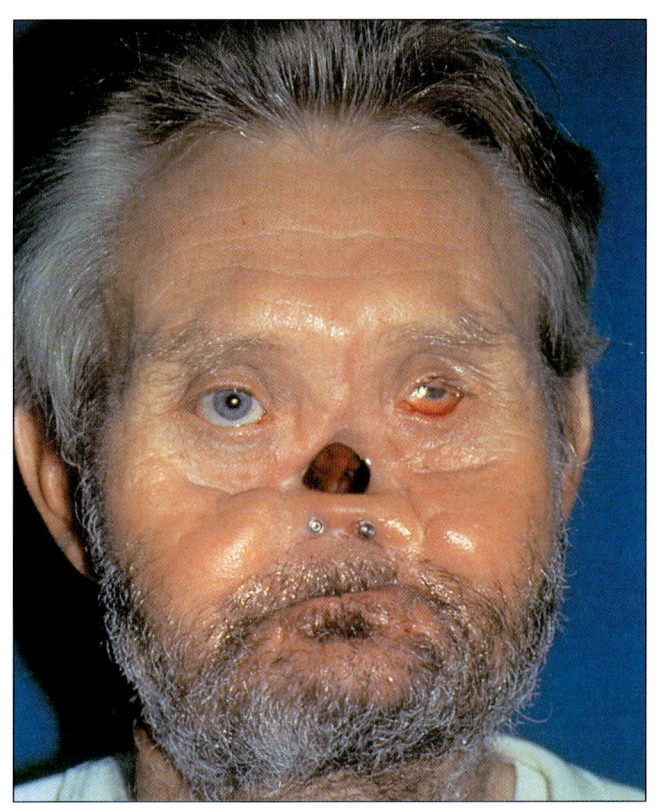
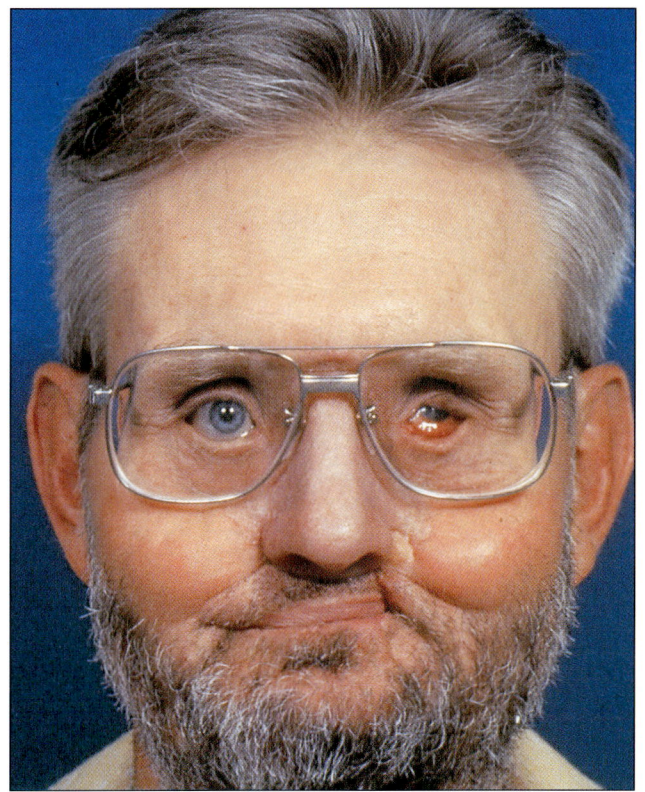
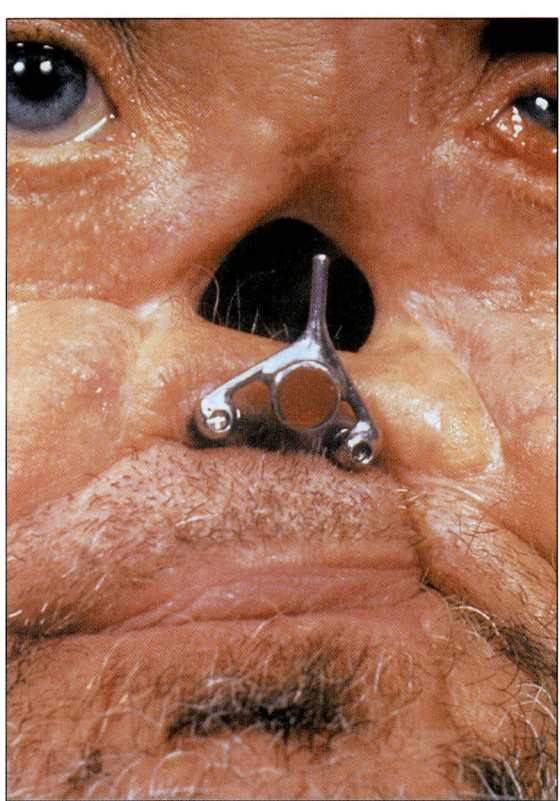
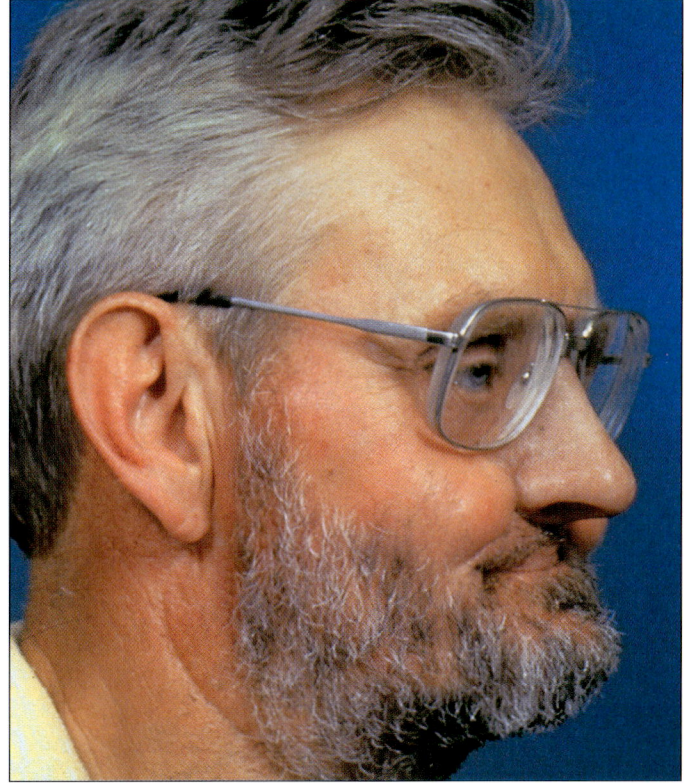

Patient Presentation 2

2 *This 61-year-old woman underwent an en bloc resection of the nose and anterior maxilla due to squamous cell carcinoma of the nasal floor at the age of 57. She was given an adhesive-retained prosthesis, that, in her opinion, did not feel secure. Two years later, five fixtures were placed in the alveolar ridge to anchor an obturator, and one fixture was placed in the nasal bone to anchor a nasal prosthesis. One month after the abutment connection, two frameworks were fabricated to anchor the prosthesis. The framework to anchor the nasal prosthesis was attached to the intraoral framework by a connection system with screws and screw-nuts. Then, a silicone nasal prosthesis was fitted onto the framework with clips. (KB)*

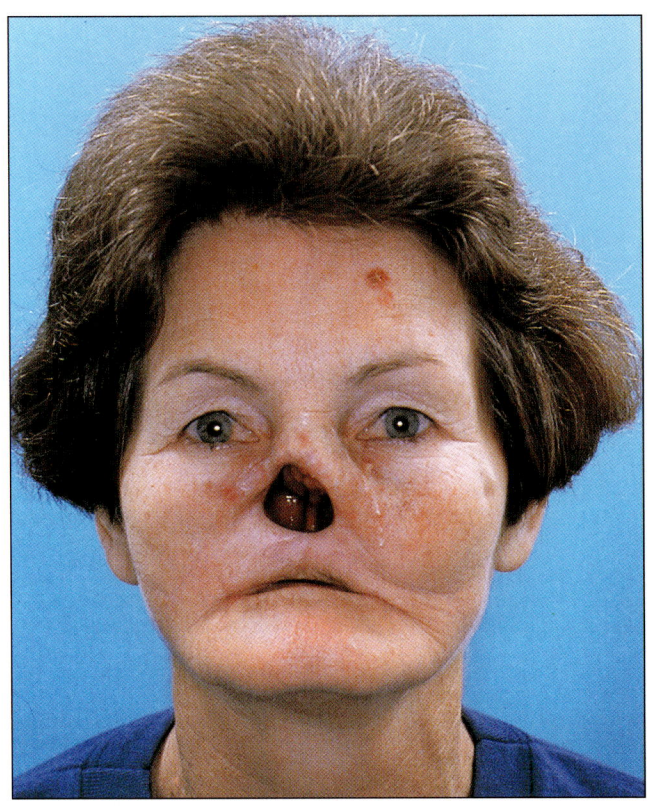
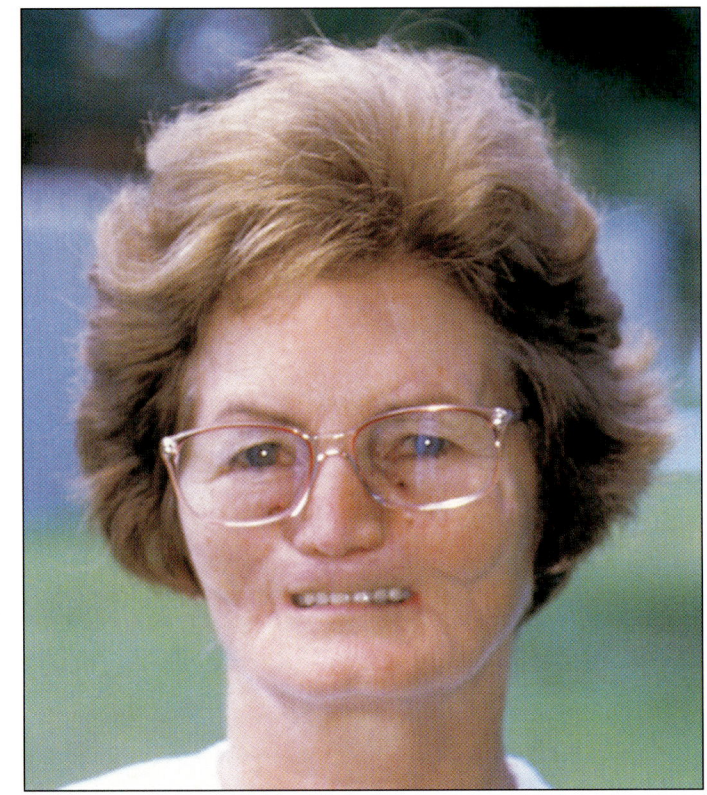
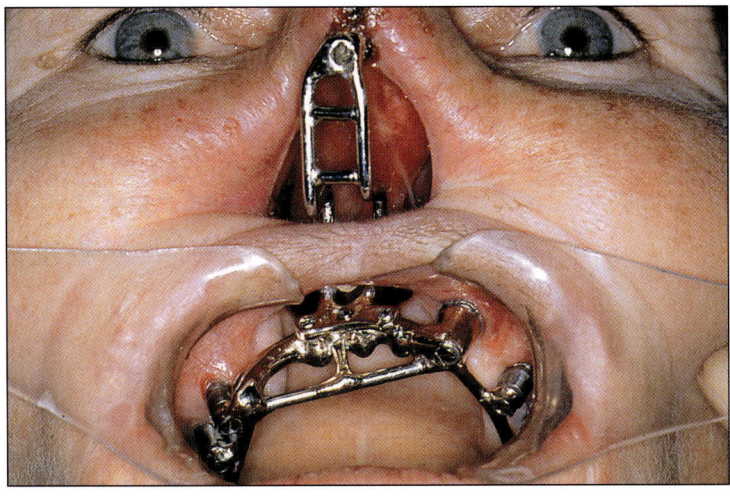
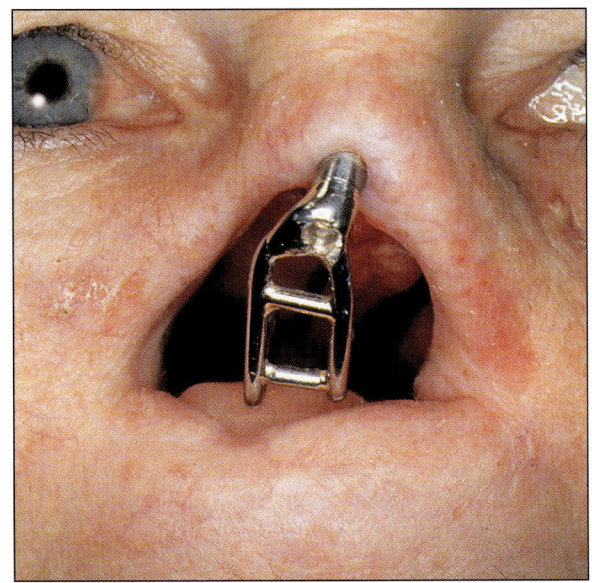

PATIENT PRESENTATION 2

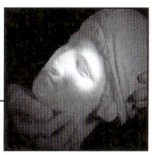

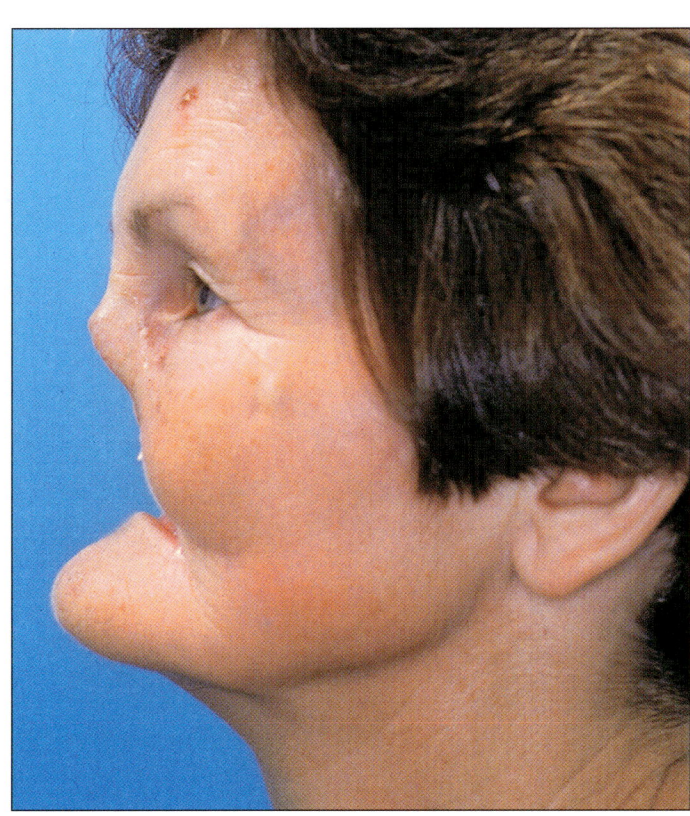

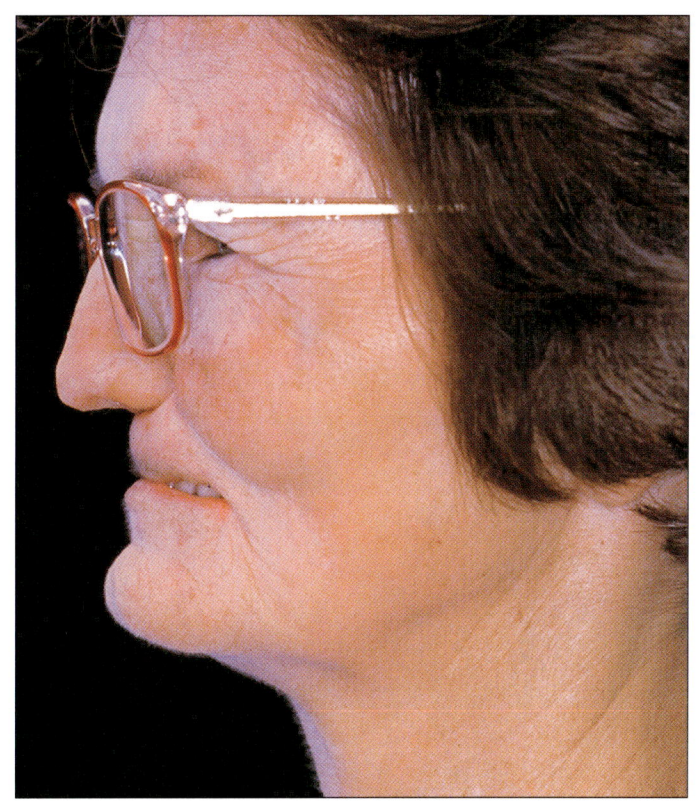

3 *This 48-year-old man underwent a left superior maxillectomy, left orbital exenteration, and total rhinectomy due to recurrent basal cell carcinoma. After the healing period, an adhesive-retained acrylic obturator was fabricated with magnetic articulation to aid retention for the silicone facial prosthesis. (AF)*

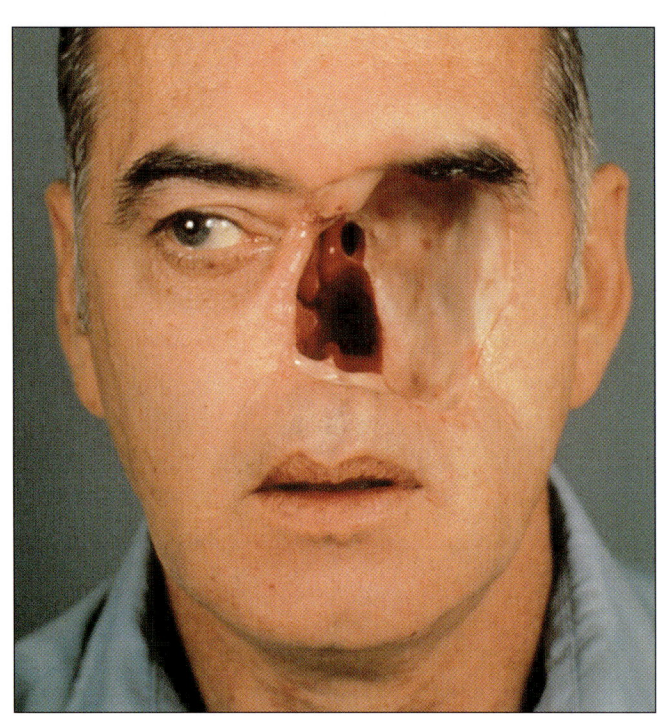
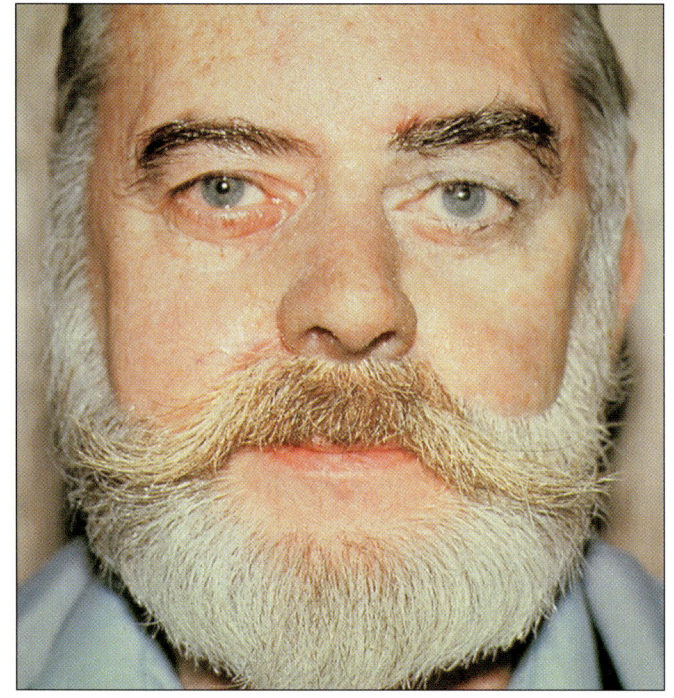
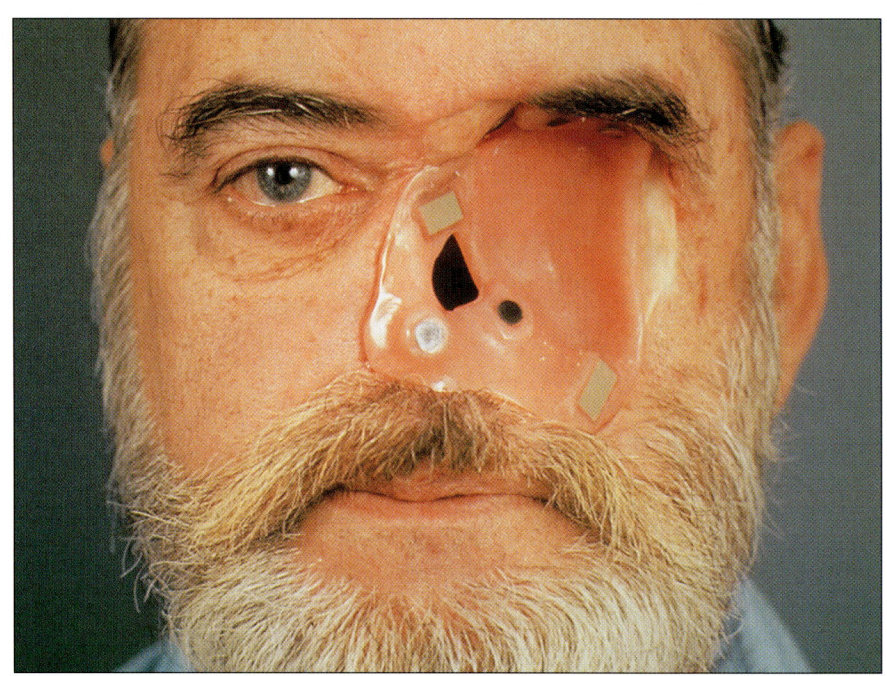

PATIENT PRESENTATION 3

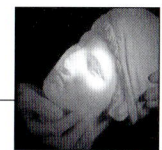

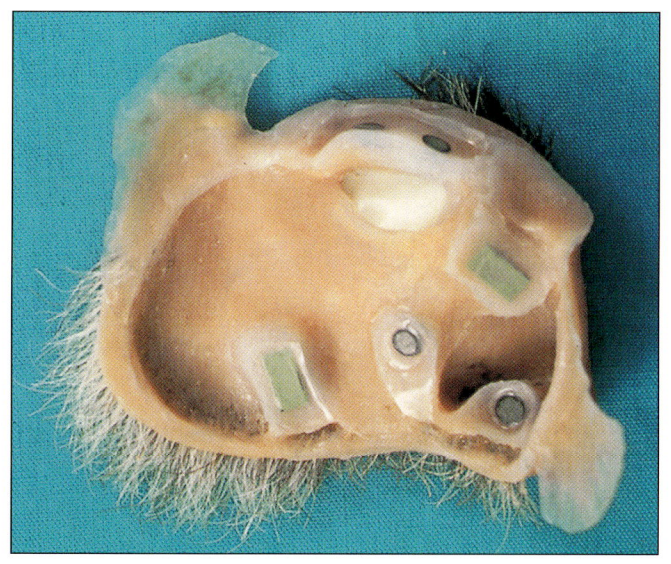

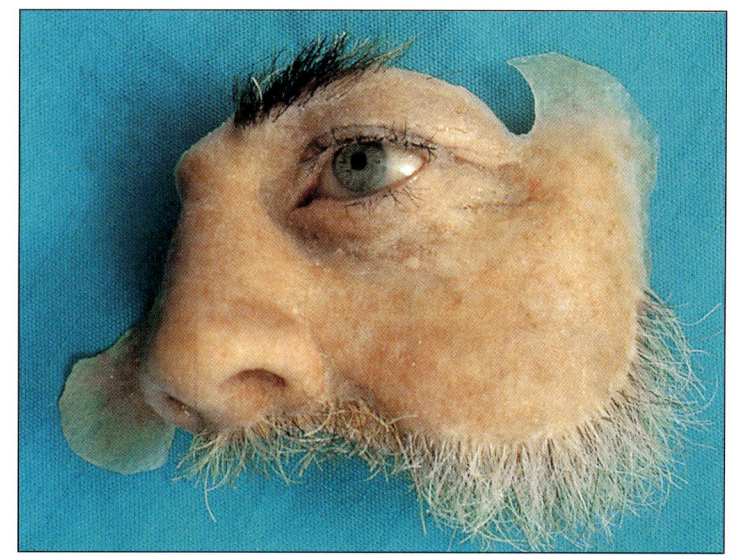

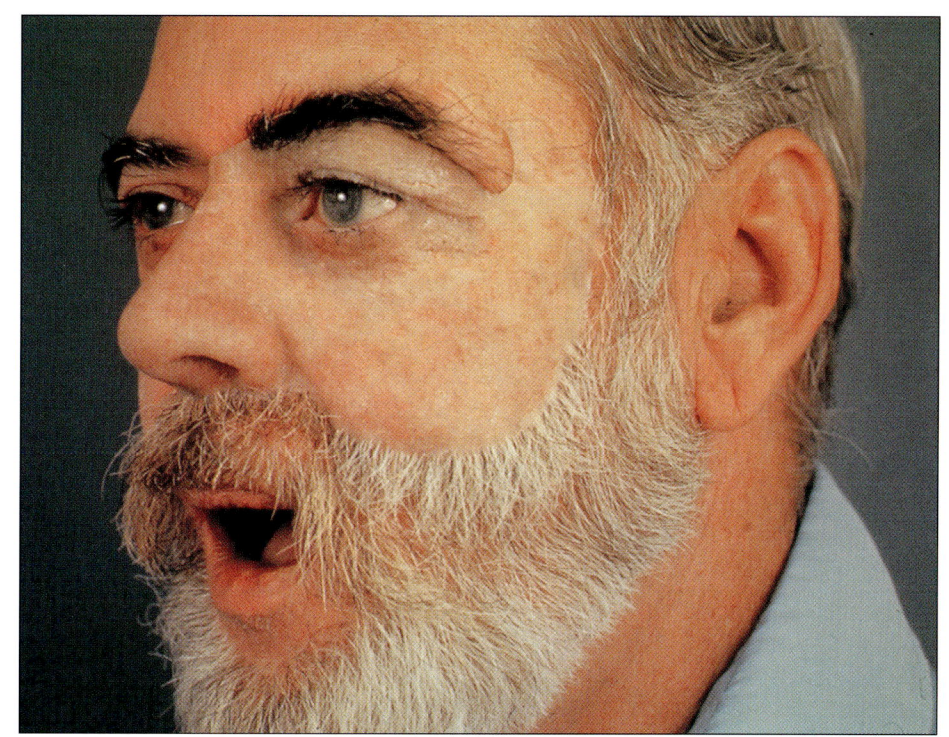

Patient Presentation 4

4 This young man was burned in a motor vehicle accident, and the injury resulted in the loss of his external ear with a wide area of alopecia. The patient history revealed that an attempt had been made to use a tissue expander to advance the hair-bearing scalp into the area of alopecia. This had been unsuccessful and the patient was unwilling to consider further tissue expansion. Fixtures were placed into the mastoid region for an auricular prosthesis, and at the same time four fixtures were placed into the cranium for an implant-retained hair-bearing prosthesis. (JW)

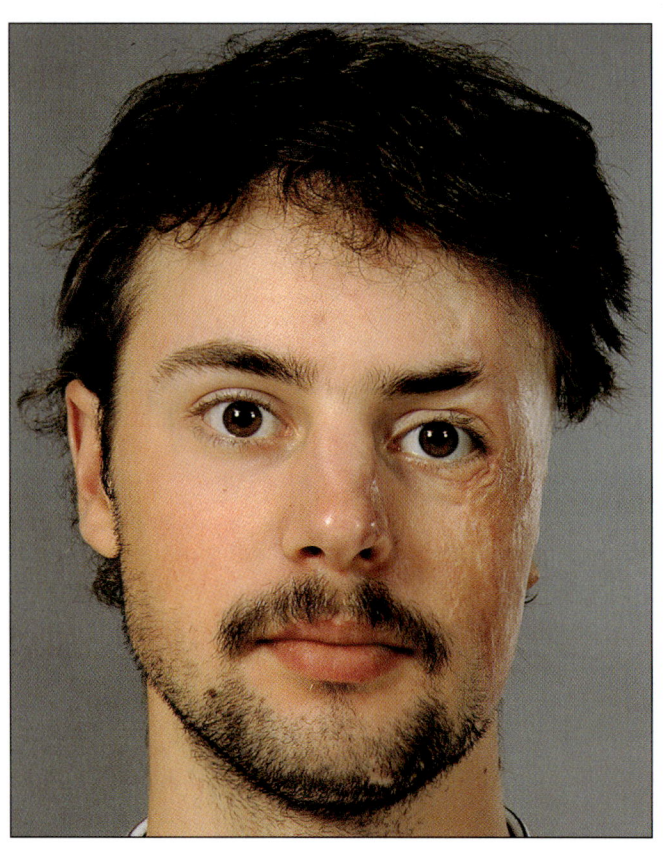
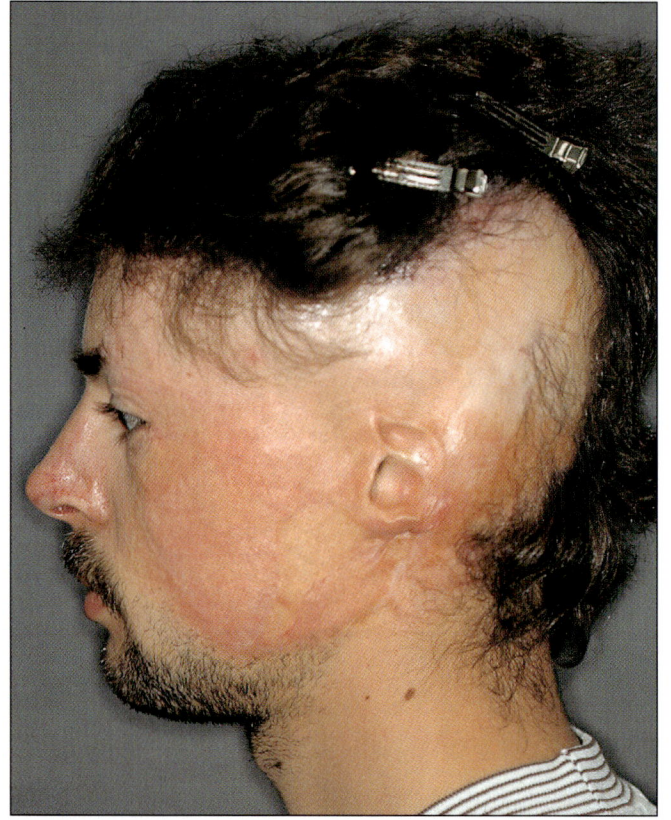
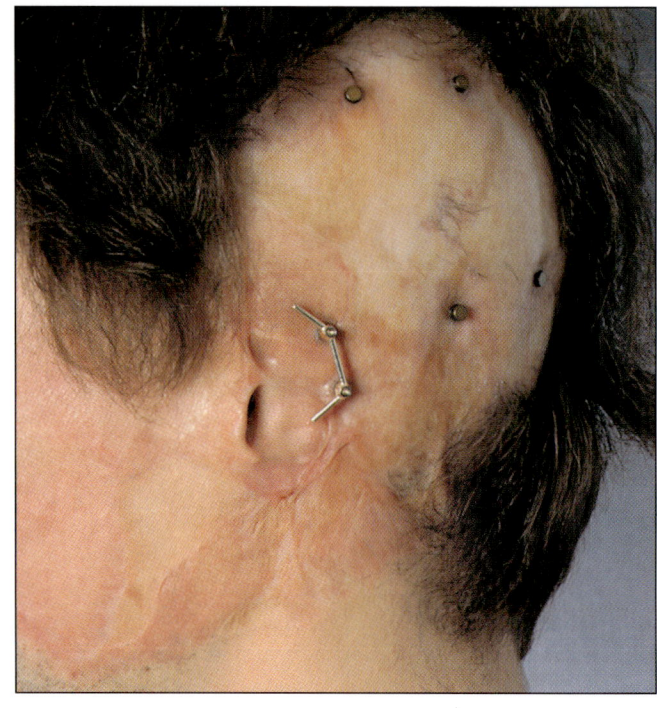

PATIENT PRESENTATION 4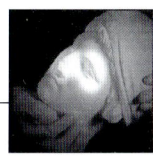

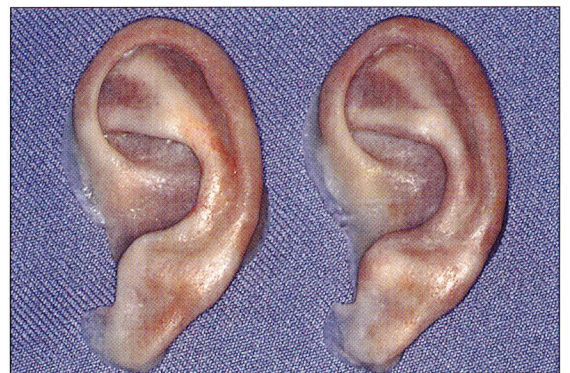
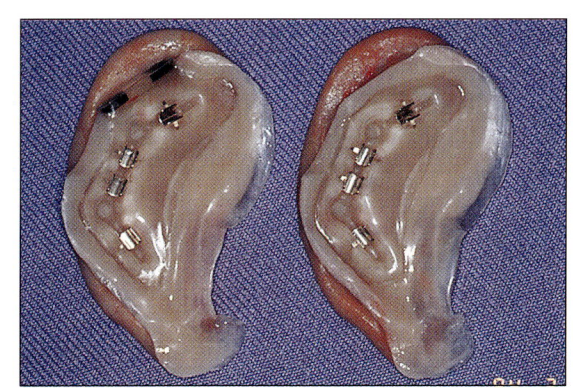
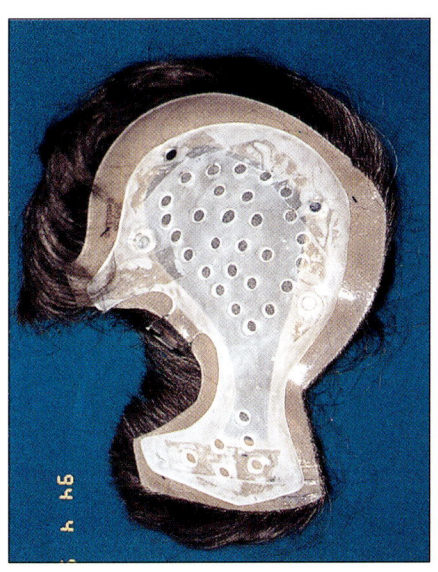
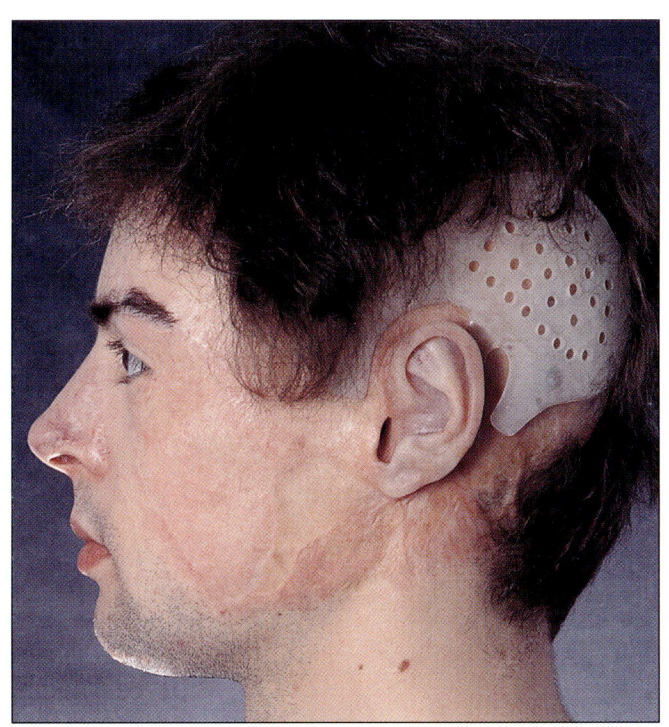
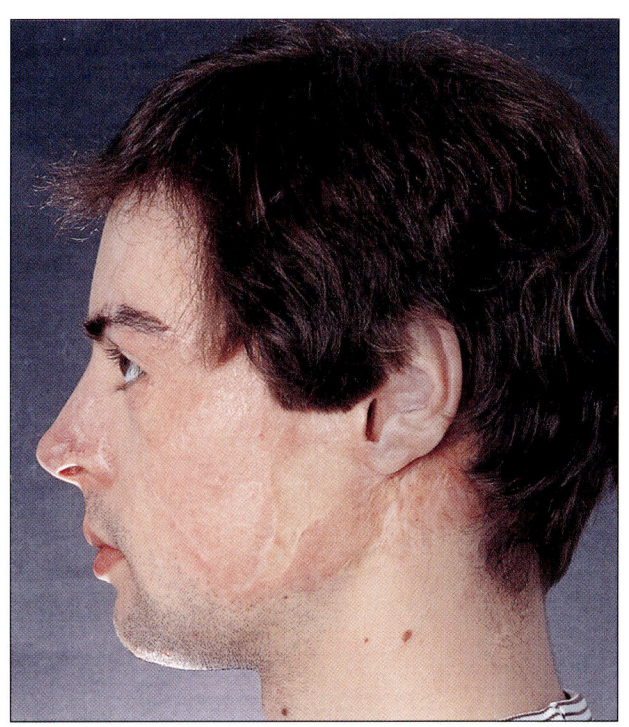

Patient Presentation 5

5 *This 77-year-old man underwent wide resection for a basal cell carcinoma, which included left orbital exenteration and partial left nasal resection. Four fixtures were placed into the supraorbital rim and maxillary area. At the second-stage procedure, console abutments were connected to the four fixtures, providing magnetic retention for the prosthesis. The selection of this method of retention was governed by the requirement that a simple path of placement be achieved. (JW)*

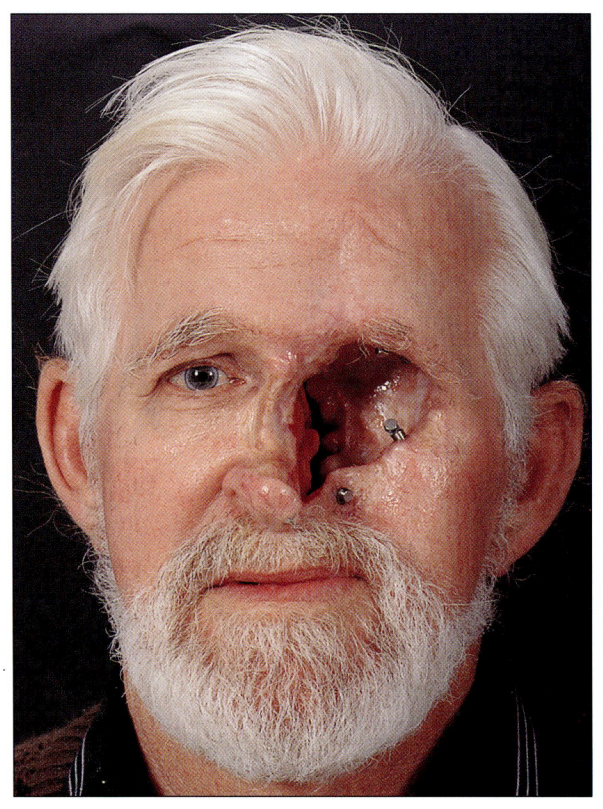
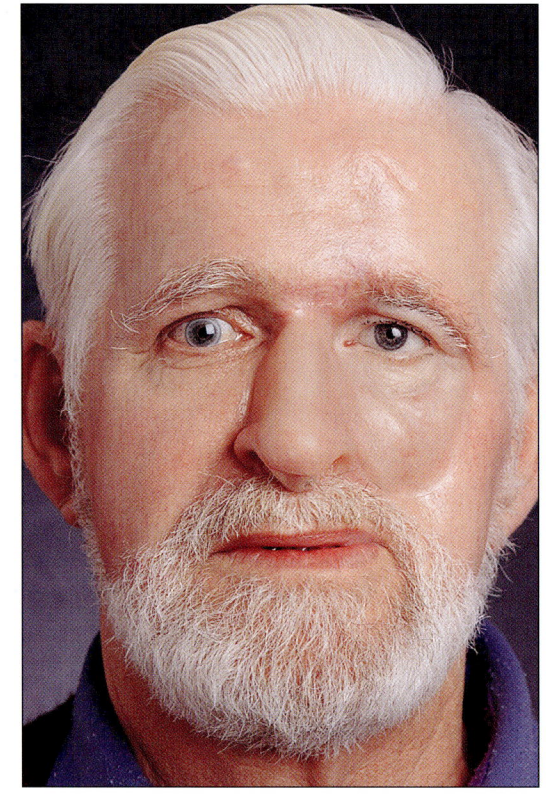
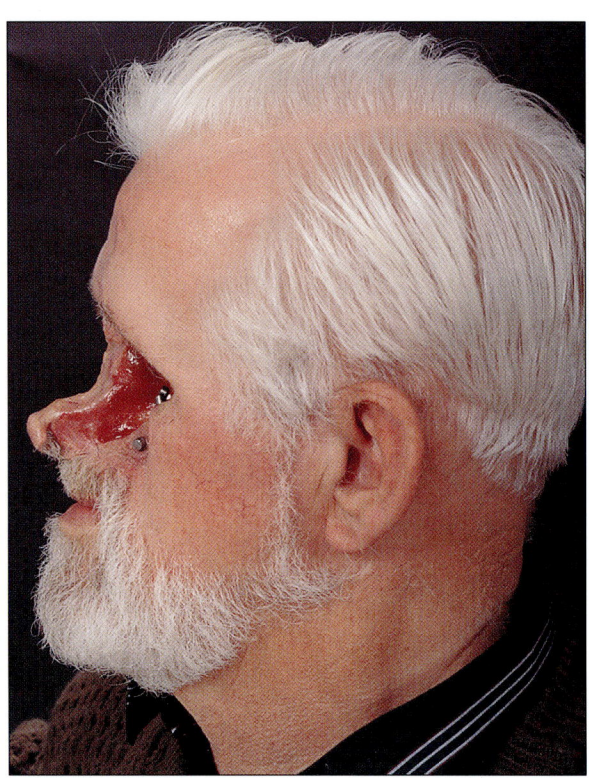
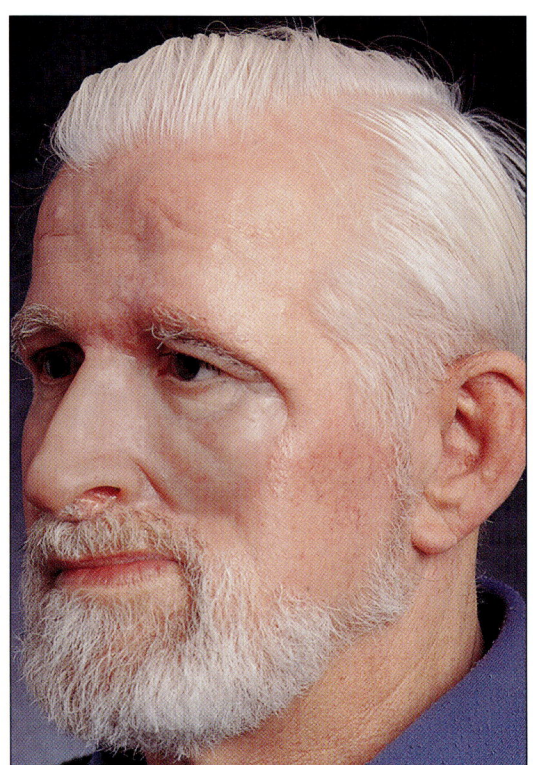

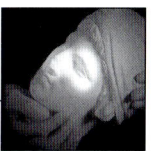
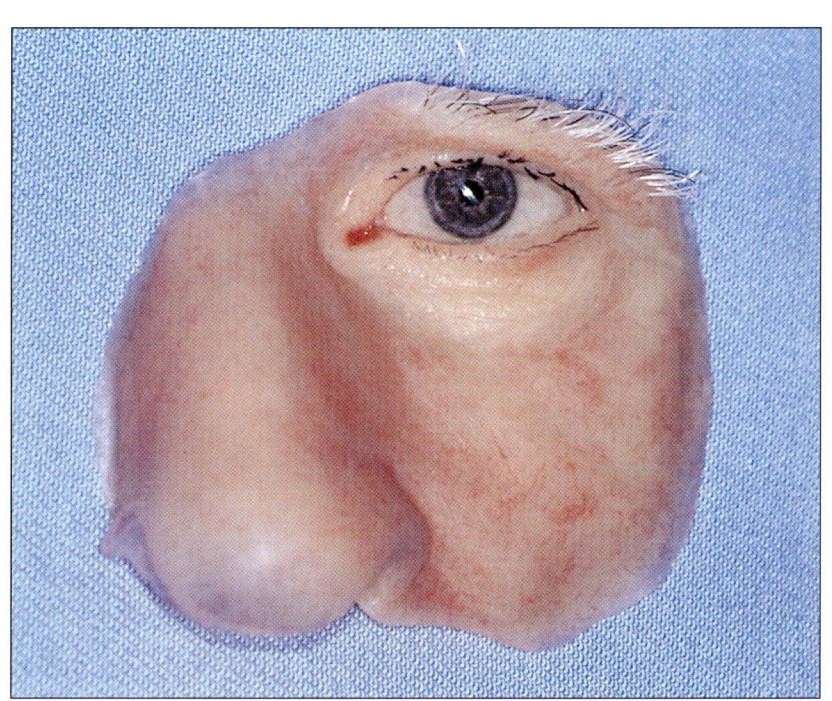
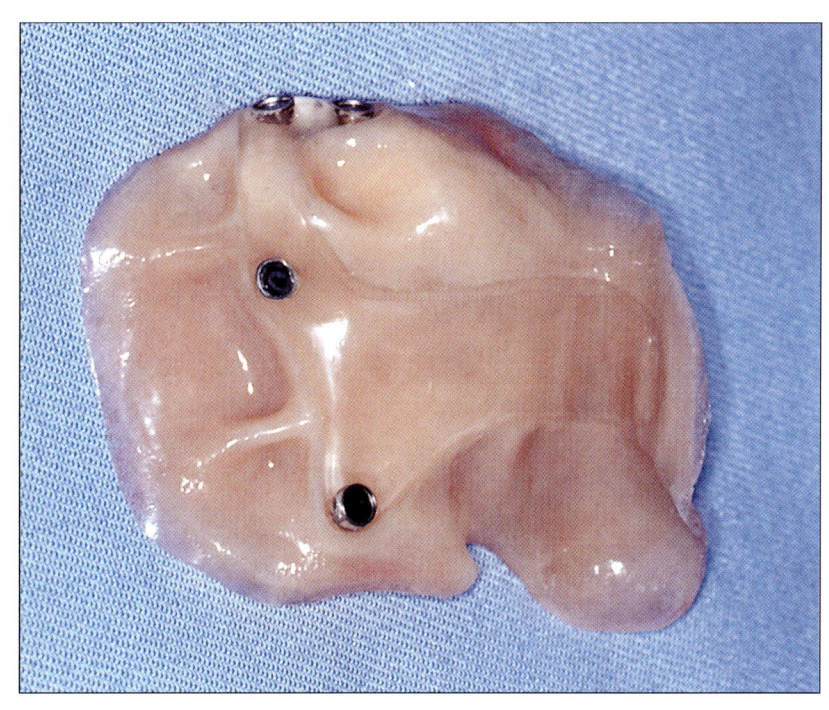

6 *This 60-year-old man underwent a left orbital exenteration with partial maxillectomy due to lymphosarcoma in 1975. The facial prosthesis was retained with adhesive and acrylic buttons placed on the upper surface of the obturator. In 1993, four extraoral fixtures were placed. After the second-stage procedure, magnets were placed onto the abutments, and the facial prosthesis was fabricated with a thin acrylic substructure to support the magnetic retention system and to prevent the formation of* Candida albicans *on the posterior surface of the prosthesis. (SH)*

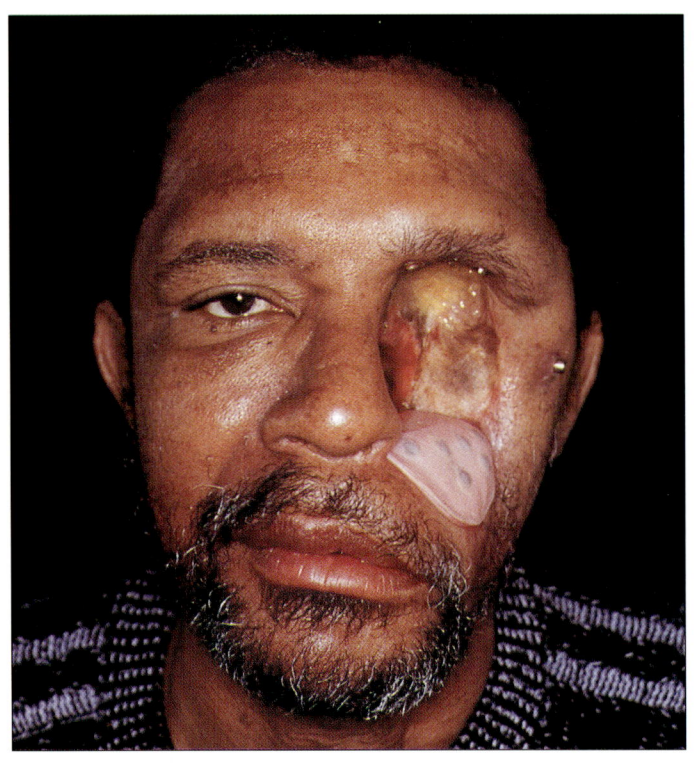
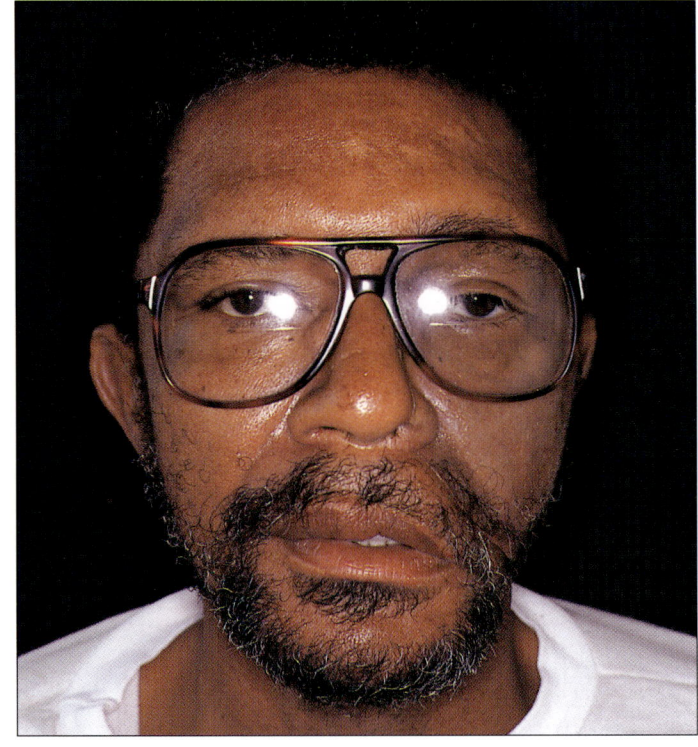
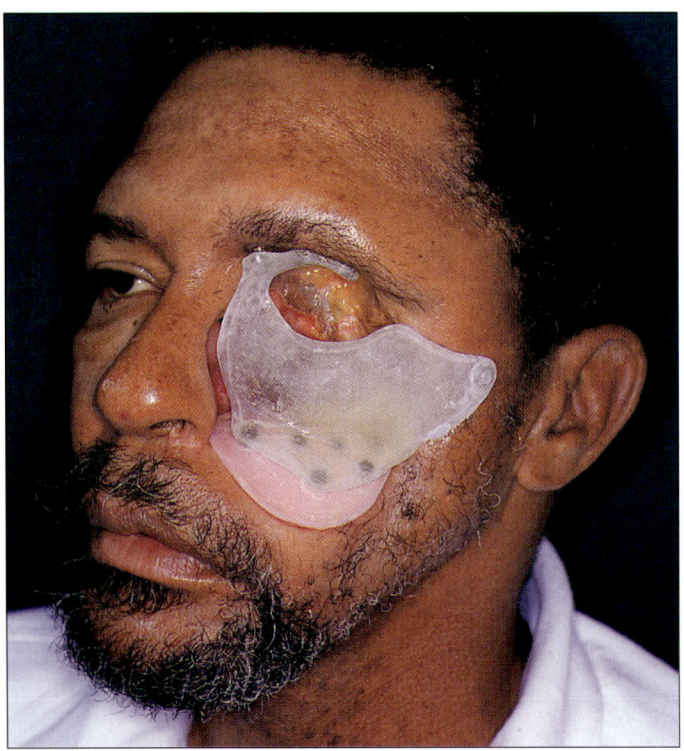
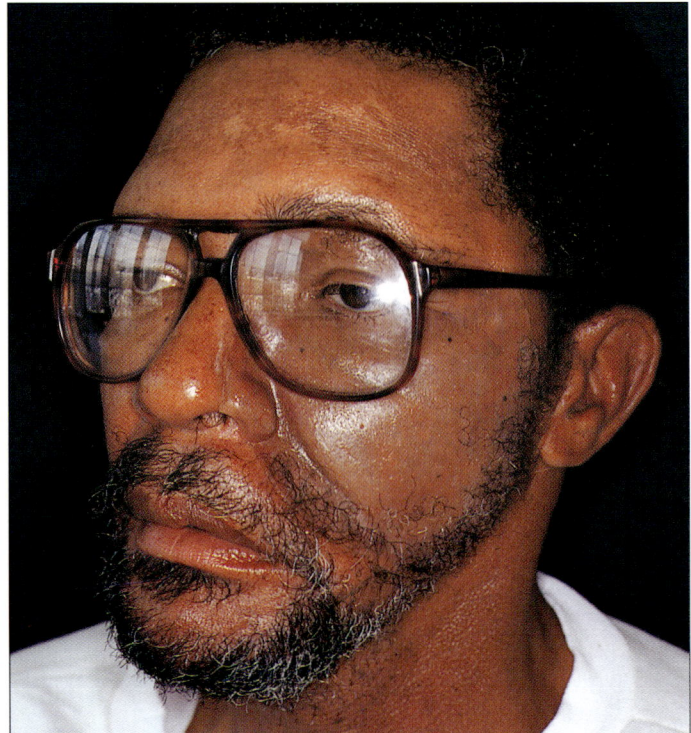

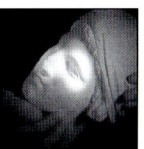

PATIENT PRESENTATION 6

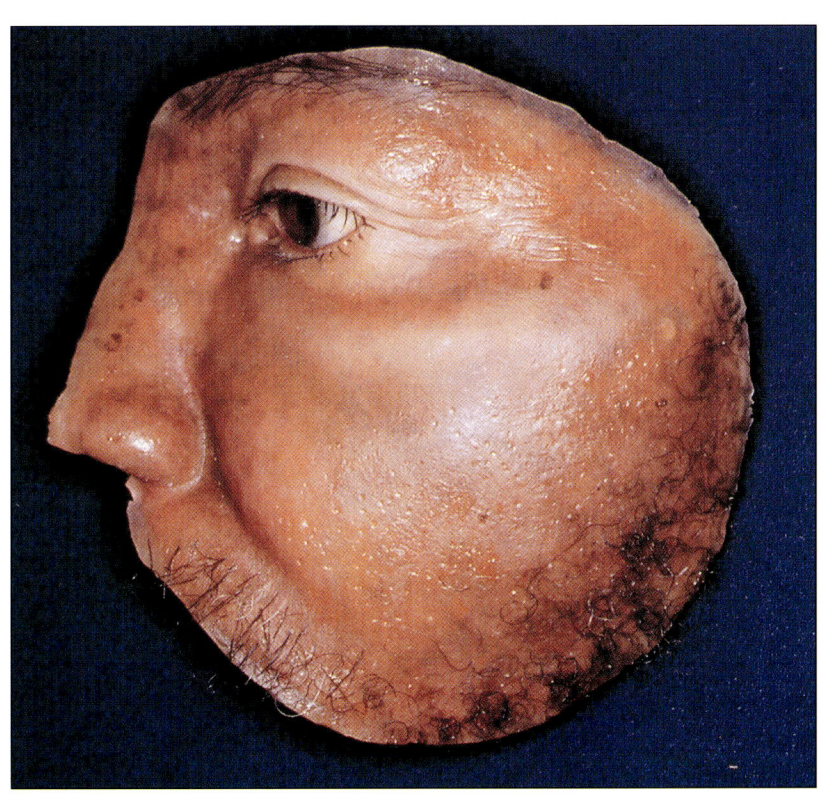
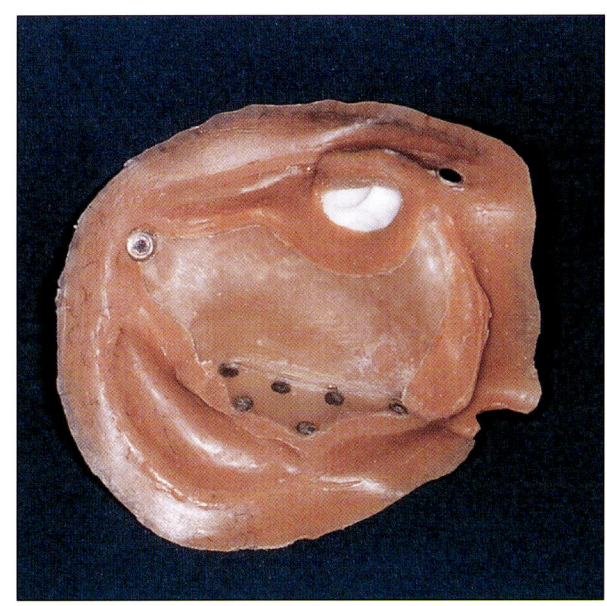

79

PATIENT PRESENTATION 7

7 *This 40-year-old woman has severe facial disfigurement suffered in a car accident. Several plastic surgical procedures were performed, but, due to the severity of her injuries, a normal appearance could not be achieved. At a later stage, seven osseointegrated implants were placed: four in the frontal bone, two in the right orbital rim, and one in the left orbital rim. A bar was later fabricated onto the abutments and the facial prosthesis was retained by 12 gold clips. (ED)*

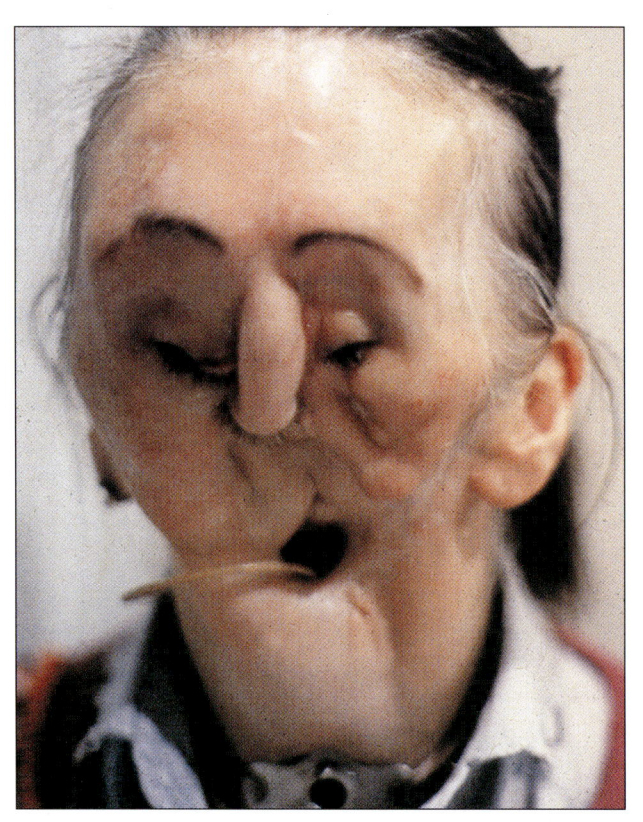
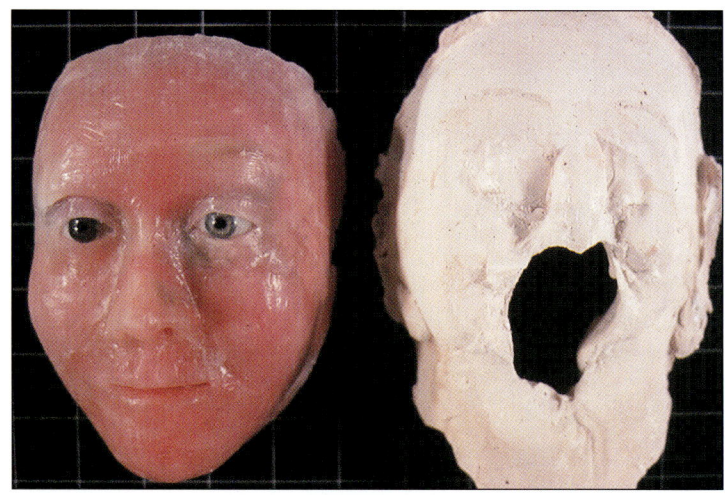
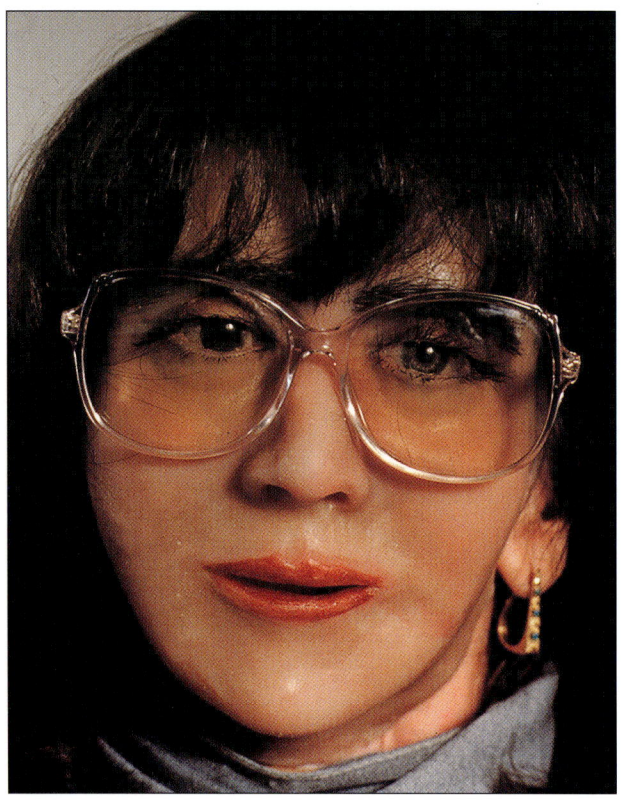
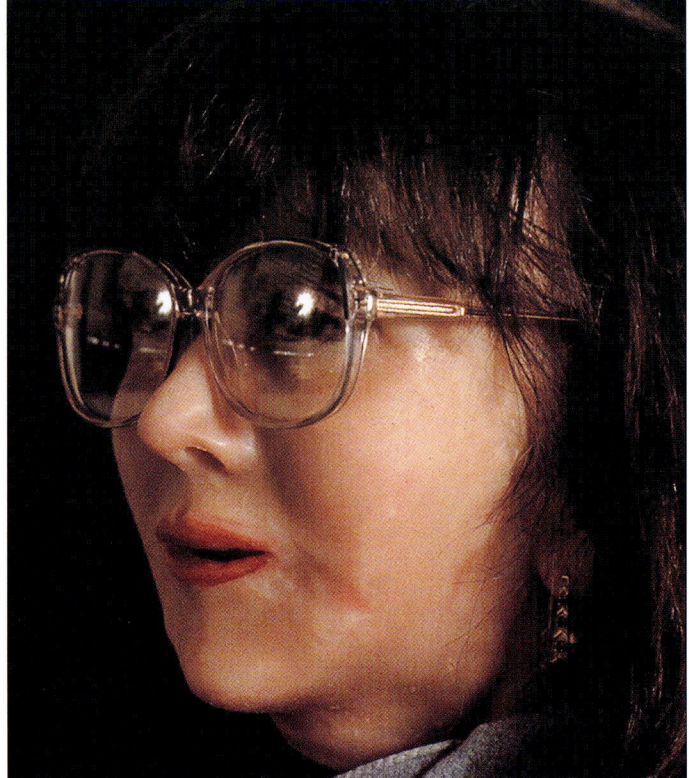

Patient Presentation 8

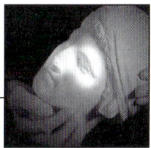

8 *This 54-year-old man suffered extensive facial injuries when he was attacked by two pit-bull terrier dogs in 1991. He underwent plastic surgery for the closure of primary defects. He was provided with a nasal prosthesis retained on glasses, but retention was poor because of ear loss and no nasal bridge. The patient was not considered a candidate for surgical reconstruction owing to extensive facial scarring. In December of the same year, two 10-mm fixtures were placed at the margins of the nasal floor, three (two of 4 mm and one of 3 mm) around the nasal bridge, and two in the mastoid. At the abutment connection, two fixtures placed in the nasal bridge were kept in reserve. In May 1992, both auricular and nasal prostheses were fitted onto two gold bars with clips. (SW)*

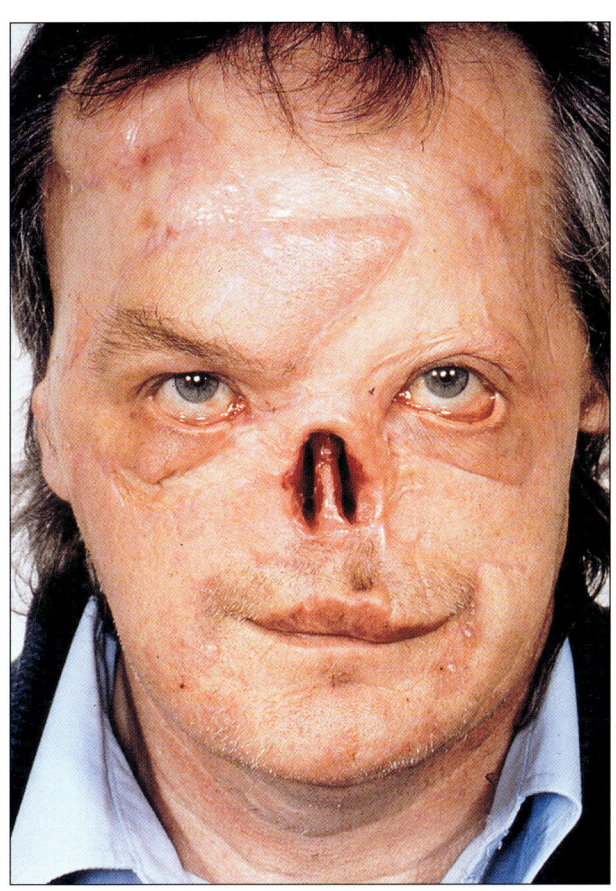
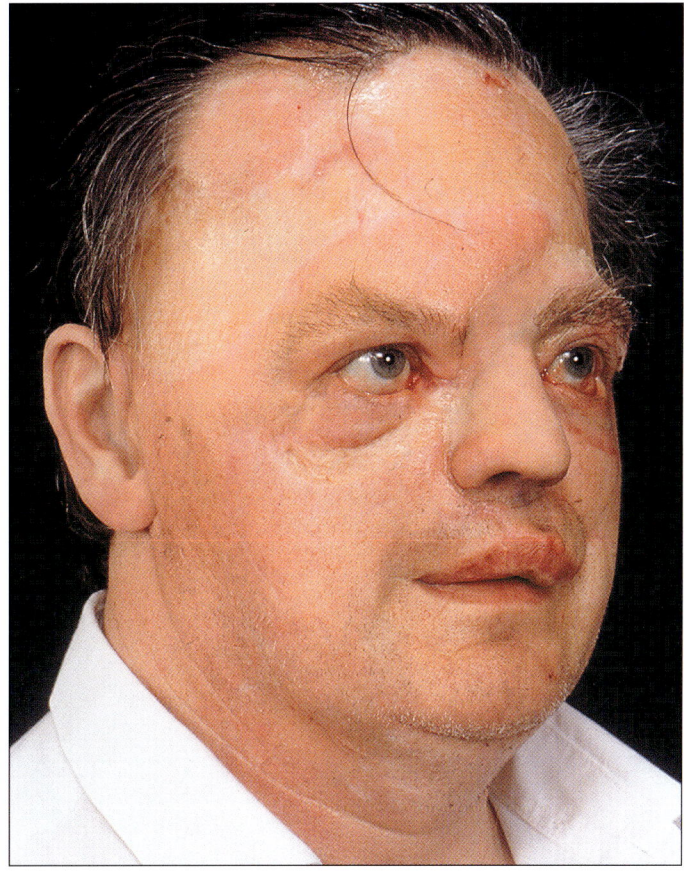

(continued)

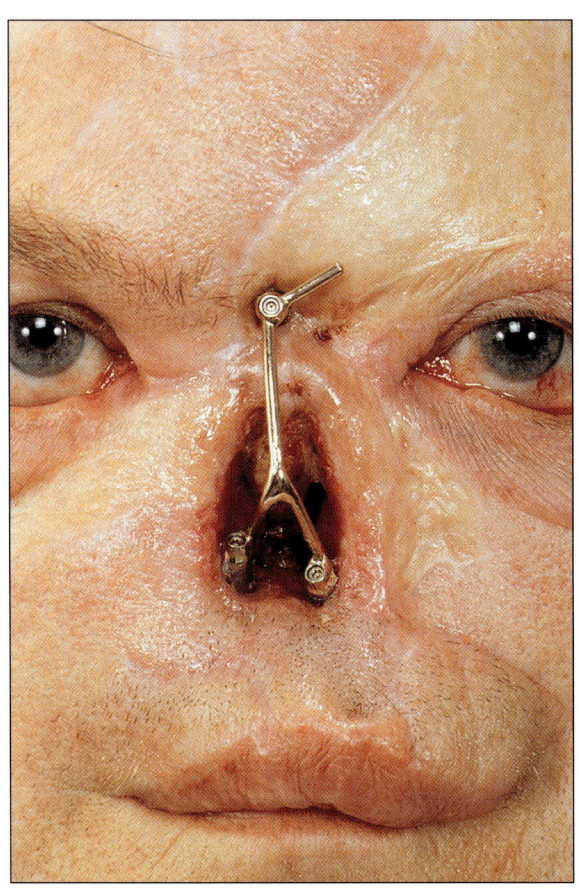
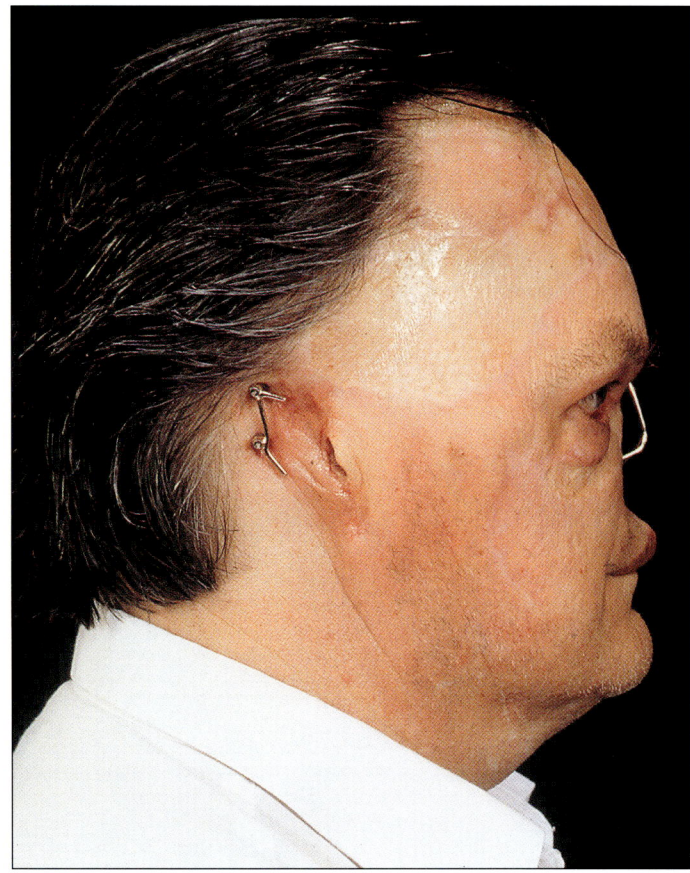
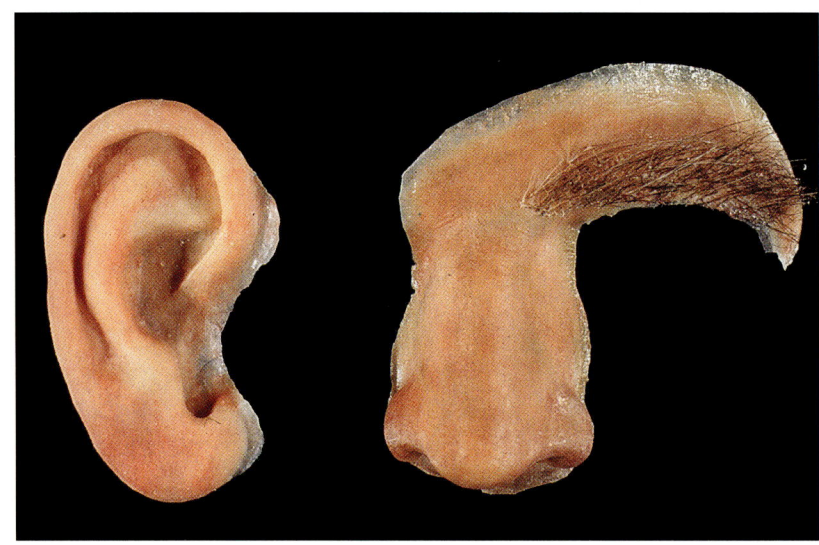

Part II
Osseointegration: Anchorage of Craniofacial Prostheses

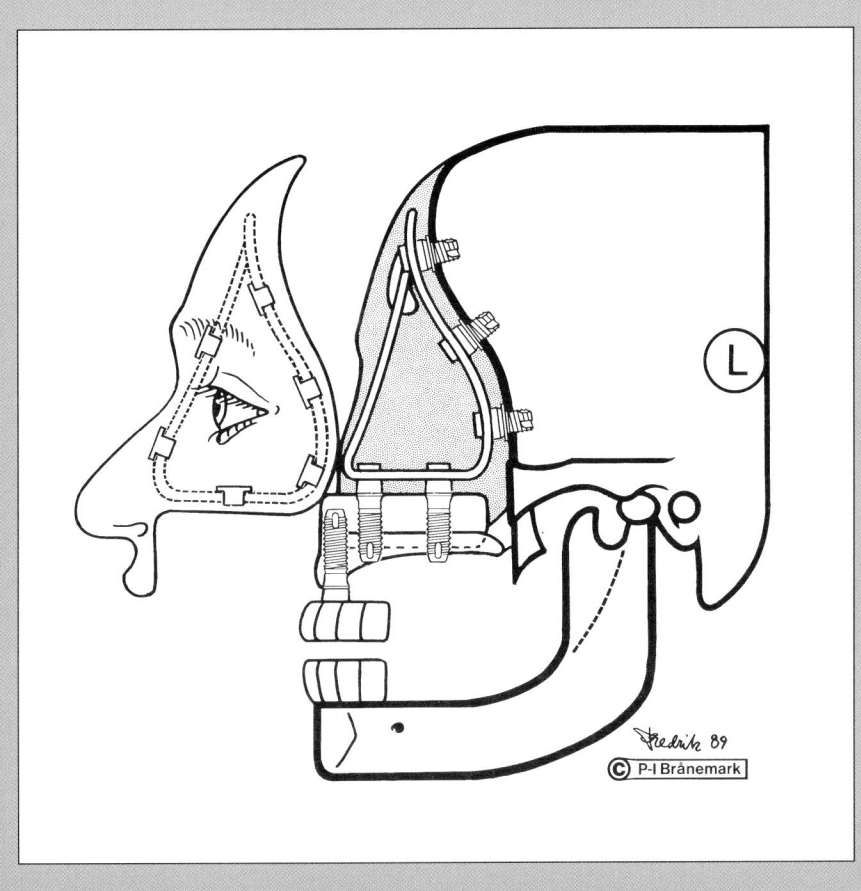

Introduction

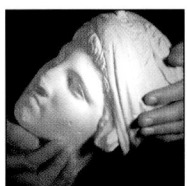

Per-Ingvar Brånemark

Ever since osseointegration was introduced as a clinical treatment option, we have participated in efforts to provide rehabilitation to patients who have craniomaxillofacial defects as a consequence of therapeutic oncologic procedures. Our clinical experience from collaborative ventures in different parts of the world indicates that these patients often present a complex treatment challenge that requires interdisciplinary preoperative, perioperative, and postoperative cooperation between patients and treatment providers (Ottawa Seminar, 1993).

If in addition to surgery, radiation therapy is provided, the vitality of hard and soft tissues is compromised, initiating a continuing pathologic process that leads to increasing problems over decades. Microvascular dysfunction and interference with metabolism and remodeling of mineralized and nonmineralized tissue are frequent sequelae of radiation therapy. In addition, impaired healing capacity affects the prognosis for reconstructive surgical procedures. A typical example of a serious complication is osteoradionecrosis.

Furthermore, if the patient or the patient's relatives cannot understand or accept the anatomic and physiologic abnormalities that oncologic procedures can cause, confidence and trust cannot be established. Even worse, if in a case of cancer that could not be radically removed, the inescapable prognostic perspectives are transferred onto health-care providers, and further professional care for such a patient becomes almost impossible.

Because of such complexities, it is reasonable that these patients are treated at special centers where the different disciplines can collaborate and where there is a wealth of experience on the selection and application of various treatment options. These centers are also valuable in the handling of unavoidable problems and complications to achieve the best possible radical or palliative result for the patient based on controlled compassion and mutual respect.

Psychiatric consultation and treatment should be considered for these patients, especially for those with head and neck tumors, because of the possible psychosocial consequences as well as more strictly medical considerations. Consultations may also be useful for concerned or involved relatives.

Craniomaxillofacial Rehabilitation in Oncology Patients

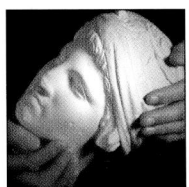

PHILIP WORTHINGTON

THE REHABILITATION OF THE CANCER PATIENT, regardless of the site of the original tumor, presents complicated problems. Nowhere is this more evident than in the case of the patient with malignant disease of the jaws and face requiring extensive surgical excision, possibly with radiation to follow.

Not exactly overlooked, but frequently underrated, is the profound psychological impact of such disease and its treatment. The face is the patient's contact with the world, and it forms the physical basis for personal recognition. Without it, the patient is robbed of his or her persona; the rapport between patient and relatives and friends, so vital to the patient's well-being, may be seriously damaged. It follows that reconstruction of the face—by whatever means—is crucial to the patient's ability to function in society, to preserve dignity, and to survive.

Certain philosophical questions arise. When the prognosis is in any way doubtful—or worse—how far should one go in providing some form of reconstruction? Some sort of balance must be reached between instilling hope and confidence on one hand and clinical reality on the other. Dealing with the patient who has a terminal disease is one thing; managing the patient who stands a fair chance of recurrent disease within 3 to 5 years is another. For the latter, what one might call palliative reconstruction can be worthwhile. This calls for sensitive judgment in each individual case.

Beyond the psychological aspect, the complexity of the structural and functional impairment is often such as to challenge the most innovative clinician. From an anatomic point of view, the patient may have lost bone, teeth, mucosa and skin, nerves, muscles, and salivary glands, perhaps the nose and/or one eye—a scene of local devastation. Function may be comparably limited. Mouth opening may be greatly restricted, the mouth may be dry, the jaws discontinuous, fistulae present, and mastication impossible. The external appearance may be shocking—at least to the lay person (Fig 1-1).

While we may agree that the radicality of the ablation should not be compromised by concern for reconstruction, the ablative surgeon should nevertheless recognize that even minimal tissue preservation may greatly facilitate reconstruction—

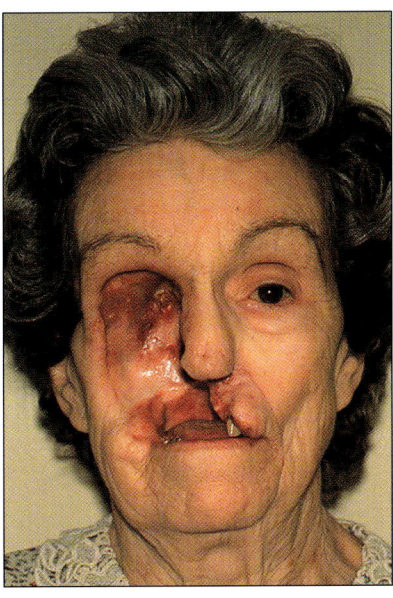

Fig 1-1 Case 1: Resection of orbit, maxilla, and upper lip leaves a severly deformed facial appearance that is deeply disturbing to the patient's friends and family.

particularly implant-supported reconstruction. There may be a choice between reconstruction using biologic tissue and a prosthetic reconstruction supported by osseointegrated implants. Both have their advantages and disadvantages. It should be remembered, however, that both methods can be combined, osseointegrated implants being installed in grafted bone, perhaps followed by free vascularized tissue transfer. Where ablation and reconstruction are performed by different surgeons, there is a paramount need for free and full communication between the two. Indeed, the difficulties of the situation frequently demand the combined talents of a true team—surgeons, nurses, prosthodontist, anaplastologist, and bioengineer.

Prosthetic reconstruction based on osseointegrated implants offers some advantages but makes certain demands. The surgical burden for the patient is commonly minor; the anchorage units provide retention and stability for the prosthesis and allow a choice between a fixed and a removable prosthesis; and access for inspection of the original operative site is preserved—most important when there is any question about the adequacy of the excision. In the case of the oral cancer patient, osseointegrated implants may counteract the loss of tongue control and the loss of the normal denture-bearing area. Most importantly, however, the implants provide the necessary stimulus to the bone graft to ensure its preservation.

For osseointegrated implants to be successful, there must be bone of adequate volume and density to allow their proper placement, ie, a sufficient number of implants of adequate length and properly distributed with due regard to their alignment. The reconstructive surgeon must pay attention to issues such as the provision of reasonably thin, attached tissue around the abutments, the restoration of sulcus form, and, for intraoral implants, the use of longer-than-normal abutments to facilitate access for maintenance.

The question of the correct timing of implant placement is difficult to answer. In some cases it may be wise to delay reconstruction for a year or two following ablation, allowing time to observe any possible recurrence. In other cases, placement at the same time as ablation may be considered. Factors influencing this decision will be the overall prognosis and the likelihood that radiation will be needed.

The complexity of the problems of the maxillofacial cancer patient are well exemplified by the hemimandibulectomy patient. At the time of excision, the surgeon should retain the temporomandibular joint and the condyle if at all possible; to retain the posterior border of the ascending ramus is often an advantage. If reconstruction is to be delayed, the jaw fragments should be stabilized in their correct spatial relationships. Most important of all, when the mandible is reconstructed, an attempt must be made to restore the mandibular volume as well as its continuity.

The residual problems of the hemimandibulectomy patient may be numerous. They may include facial deformity because of loss of bone and mandibular drifting, malocclusion and inability to chew, difficulty with speech and swallowing, possible drooling of saliva, impaired muscle control and limitation of mandibular movement, and loss of sensation in the lip or tongue or both. The available denture-bearing area is diminished, biting force is lessened, and conventional prostheses have no stability or retention. In many cases, there will be no proper vestibular or lingual sulcus form to the mucosa, and the tongue may be tethered to the cheek or mandible or lip. The soft tissue of pedicled flaps or free flaps used for immediate reconstruction may be inappropriately thick and mobile. Altogether a daunting prospect. In such circumstances, what is the role of osseointegration?

Figure 1-2 shows a patient in whom the postoperative defect extended beyond the loss of bone and teeth to include muscle, mucosa, and nerve. A carcinoma of the floor of the mouth had been irradiated and later resected. The mandible had been excised from one molar region to the other, the deficiency being restored by a bone graft (Fig 1-3). Soft-tissue cover had been provided by a combination of tongue flap and chest flap. While the details of the surgery are not important here, the end result was one of an abnormal tongue, a mandible covered by a thick and mobile layer of soft tissue, with little residual dentition and a lower lip that was insensitive (Fig 1-4).

The first step was to thin the chest flap to provide a thin, attached layer of tissue over the symphysis (Fig 1-5). Then by means of osseointegrated implants, firm anchorage was provided for a complete lower fixed bridge; in this way, the dentition was restored and the occlusion optimized (Fig 1-6). The residual problem was that the patient drooled saliva. This problem was corrected by the prosthodontist, who provided a removable silicone dam to fit against and around the abutment cylinders behind the insensitive lip (Fig 1-7). By these means, the patient was able to speak and eat again and to re-enter society.

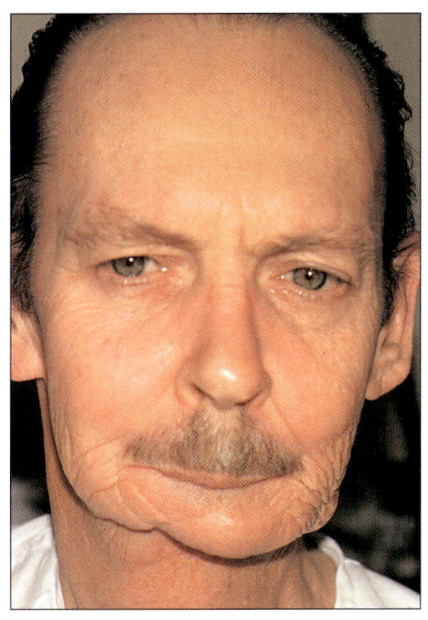

Fig 1-2 Case 2: Patient following the resection of a tumor of floor of mouth with prior irradiation.

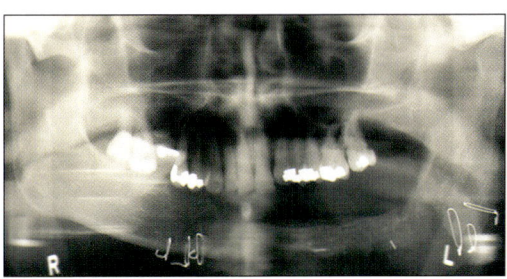

Fig 1-3 Same patient's panoramic radiograph showing bone-graft reconstruction from one premolar region to the opposite molar region.

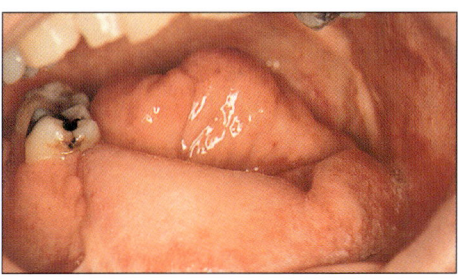

Fig 1-4 Same patient: the oral anatomy is quite abnormal following repair using a median-transit tongue flap and deltopectoral (D-P) flap for resurfacing the floor of the mouth and covering the reconstructed mandible. The D-P flap is thick and mobile over the mandible.

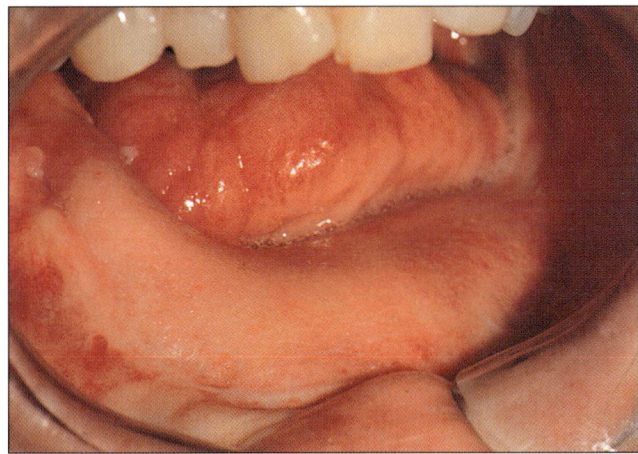

Fig 1-5 As a first step, the D-P flap is markedly thinned over the mandibular bone graft to provide tissue that is not merely thinner but somewhat tethered to the bone, thus providing attached tissue to surround the future abutments.

Fig 1-6 Satisfactory restoration of occlusion with an implant-supported bridge in lower jaw against upper natural teeth. Salivary control was difficult due to lack of sensation in the lower lip and impaired muscle function.

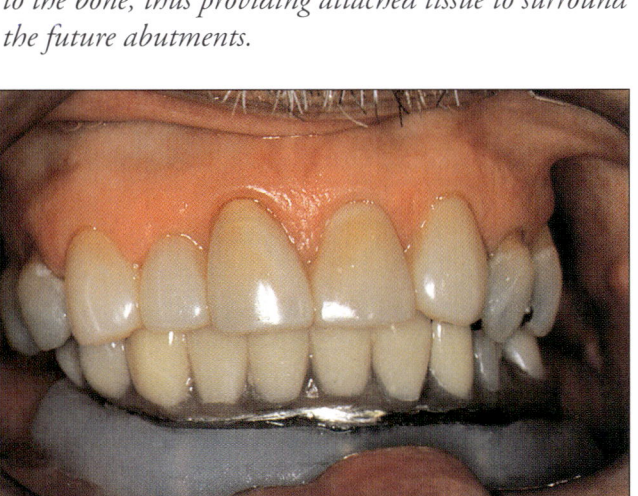

Fig 1-7 Thanks to provision of a silicone dam, fitting against and around the lower abutments, drooling was eliminated.

Following mandibular resection, a bone graft may adequately restore mandibular continuity and provide acceptable external facial contours, but rehabilitation is incomplete until the dentition and oral function are restored (Fig 1-8). In this case, four 18-mm implants were placed into the bone graft and the abutments added later.

In such cases, however, one meets with certain problems. Where the perimandibular soft tissues have been sacrificed, the oral mucosa from the tongue or lingual pouch may just touch the top of the graft and then pass vertically up the inside of the cheek with no vestige of lingual or buccal sulcus form. The consequence is difficulty in oral hygiene, irritation, and hyperplasia of the mucosa (Fig 1-9). To prevent the irritation of mobile mucosa rubbing against the abutment cylinders, one may need to place a split skin graft alongside the abutments to provide a band of attached, nonmobile tissue (Fig 1-10). In this patient, the reconstruction was then completed with a fixed bridge, and speech and mastication were vastly improved (Fig 1-11). The patient is now 12 years postresection.

The same technology and similar principles apply to various forms of maxillofacial and craniofacial reconstruction. Because of its versatility, its small surgical burden for the patient, and its minimal dependence on biologic tissues, osseointegration has taken a central role in the rehabilitation of the craniomaxillofacial oncology patient.

Fig 1-8 Case 3: (a) Satisfactory restoration of external mandibular contours following bone graft reconstruction of the mandible after resection for tumor. (b) The dentition is severely impaired by loss of almost one quadrant.

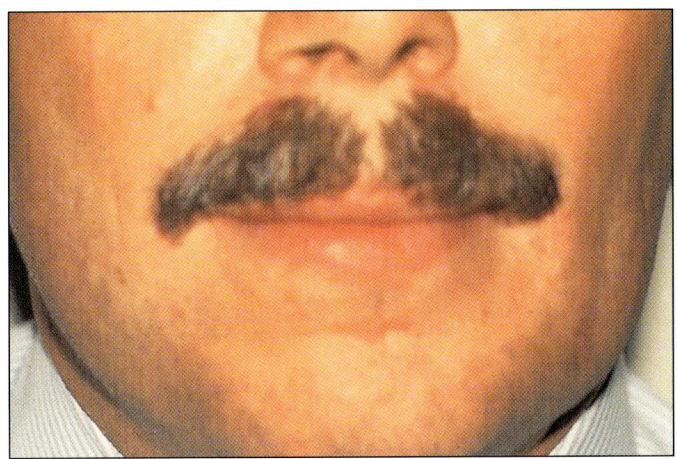

a

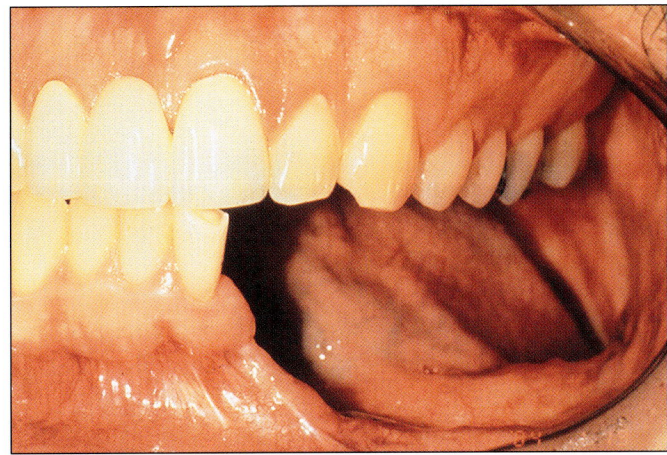

b

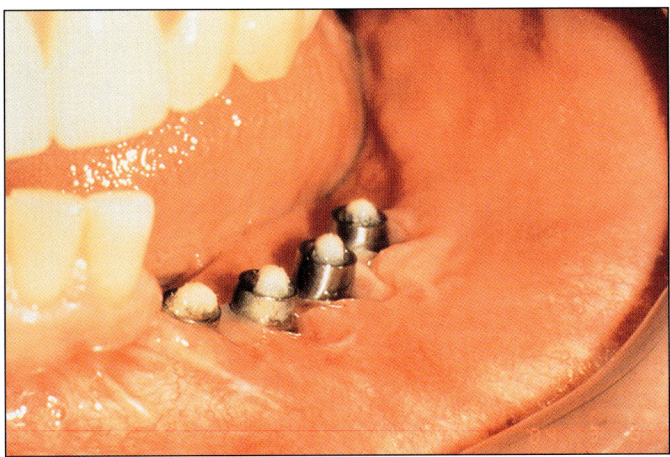

Fig 1-9 After placement of four 18-mm implants in the bone graft and addition of abutment cylinders, the residual problem is irritation of the mucosa due to the lack of attached tissue adjacent to the abutments. Oral hygiene is difficult to maintain and consequently there is a tendency to mucosal hyperplasia.

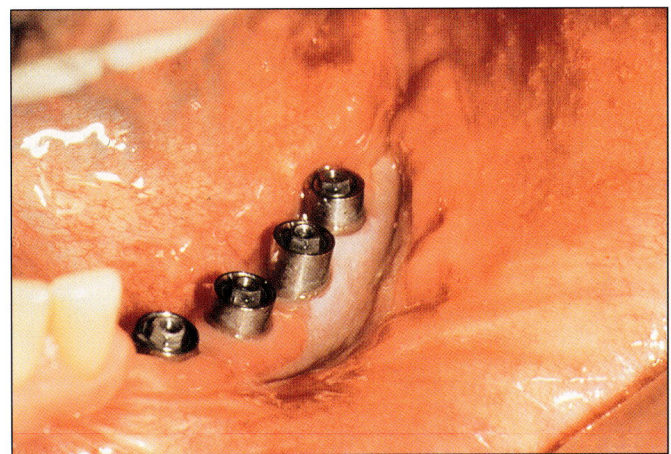

Fig 1-10 Placement of a split skin graft alongside the mandibular abutments tethers the tissue, facilitates hygiene, and eliminates the tendency to irritation and hyperplasia.

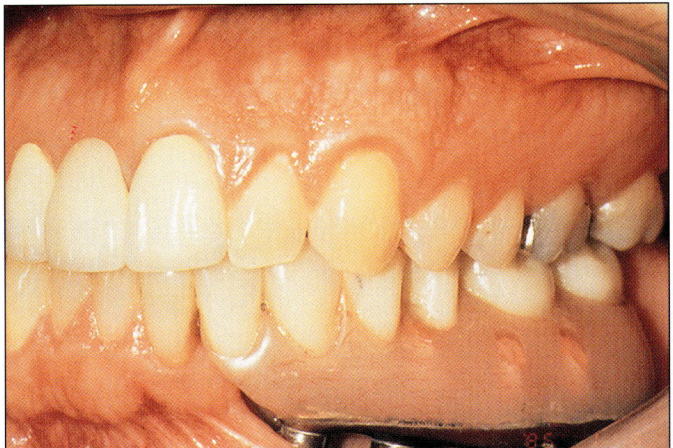

Fig 1-11 Restoration of masticatory efficiency and improvement in speech and appearance follow placement of the implant-supported prosthesis for the defective quadrant.

2

Plastic and Reconstructive Surgery

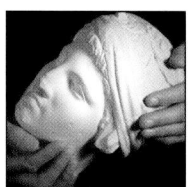

Elof Eriksson

Reconstructive craniomaxillofacial surgery has undergone a rapid evolution over the past decades. The diagnosis of various defects has been greatly aided by three-dimensional imaging techniques, such as computed tomography (CT) or magnetic resonance imaging (MRI), where these images can be used for a computer-generated image of the deformed facial skeleton.

Modern craniofacial surgery, which is usually performed through a coronal incision, has greatly expanded the possibilities of remodeling the craniofacial skeleton in a precise and predictable fashion. Microvascular free tissue transfer of flaps containing skin and sometimes muscle and bone are commonplace in the reconstruction of complex craniofacial defects from tumor ablation or trauma. Tissue expansion has also become an important technique for the reconstruction of, in particular, the hair-bearing scalp, but also other facial skin defects where it is highly desirable to use skin of similar color and texture.

Timing of Reconstruction

Craniomaxillofacial defects should be reconstructed as soon as the patient's condition is stable enough to allow the reconstructive procedures. With today's standard of care, it is no longer acceptable to leave the patient with a disfigurement that can almost always be reconstructed with either autogenous or prosthetic techniques.

In the past, some institutions have chosen to delay craniofacial reconstruction after certain procedures such as tumor ablation. The reasons for this have usually been described as a desire to rule out local recurrence of the tumor before undertaking reconstruction. With the increased sophistication in craniomaxillofacial reconstruction in combination with the safety of the various surgical procedures, delaying reconstruction is no longer necessary. Even if the patient has a life expectancy of only months to a few years, it is unacceptable for the patient to spend this time with a facial deformity that precludes a normal social and family life.

Diagnosis and Preoperative Planning

It is imperative to have a complete understanding of the three-dimensional defect to be reconstructed. Not only must the exact amount of bone and soft tissue required be known, but it is also important to know the size of the various areas that need to be covered with epithelium, as well as how far apart they are (as where, for instance, the same piece of skin is used for both the reconstruction of oral and nasal epithelium and external skin coverage). Computed tomography and MRI are very useful in the three-dimensional diagnosis of the deformities. In addition, frequently used are alginate molds, which can be incised and unfolded to illustrate what two-dimensional piece of tissue needs to be used to reconstruct a three-dimensional defect. It is also important to make the skin cover slightly too large to accommodate early postoperative swelling.

Surgical Principles and Techniques

In general, it is preferable to perform the reconstruction immediately after ablation of the tumor, or as soon as possible after the occurrence of a traumatic injury. If a sufficient amount of soft tissue is present, small hard-tissue defects can usually be reconstructed with nonvascularized bone grafts. If soft tissue is missing and the hard-tissue defect is large, vascularized bone is usually used, often as a composite flap containing bone as well as skin for the surface reconstruction. Iliac crest, fibula, scapula, and the radius are usually the preferred donor sites for this kind of reconstruction. The fixation of the reconstructed bone is very important, and plates with screws are usually the preferred method of skeletal fixation.

Small, superficial soft-tissue defects are often covered with skin grafts or composite grafts, while deeper small defects can be reconstructed with local flaps. If the soft-tissue defect is large, one usually has to use a free flap for coverage. The most useful flaps are thin with a large surface area-to-volume ratio, making them useful in both the reconstruction of intraoral as well as extraoral defects. In this situation, the radial forearm flap is often used.

Localized defects of the scalp in the presence of good hair growth in the intact part of the scalp make tissue expansion a useful modality for scalp reconstruction. The expander, which consists of an empty silicone balloon with a subcutaneous injection port, is placed underneath an area of intact scalp. Saline is then injected once or twice weekly into the expander, which will stretch the intact scalp or skin until a sufficient amount is available for coverage of the defect. In this fashion, large scalp defects as well as facial and neck defects can be reconstructed. In certain areas, particularly the eyelids and the nose, local flaps are preferred because of their color, texture, and thinness.

Fig 2-1 This 61-year-old man sustained a deep facial burn resulting in the loss of most of his nose 2 weeks previously (a). As a first stage of the nasal reconstruction, a flap based on his radial artery and cephalic vein is prepared on his arm with cartilage grafts to the nasal tip and ala and skin grafts for the lining of his nostrils (b). The flap was also designed to provide skin cover over his cheek. Six months after transfer of the flap, frontal view (c) and lateral view (d) show an acceptable autogenous reconstruction of his nose. (Treatment by Dr Julian Pribaz and the author.)

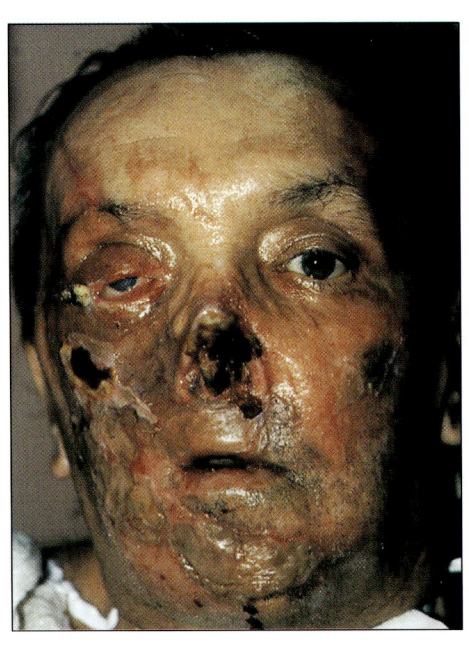

a

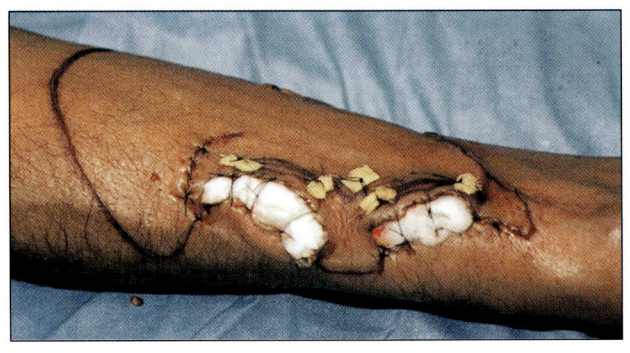

b

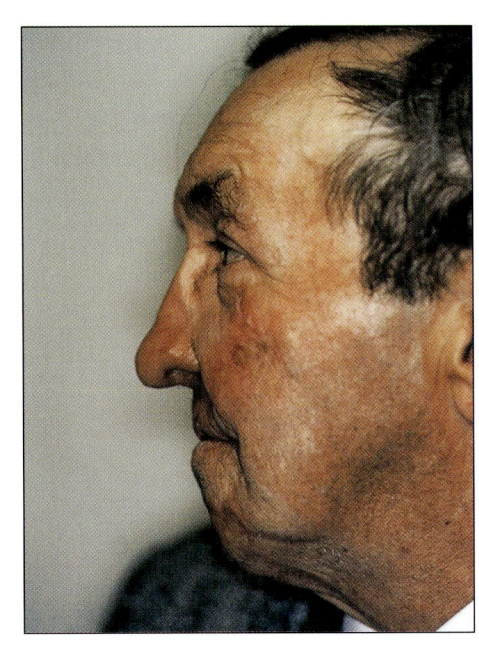

c

d

Autogenous vs Prosthetic Reconstruction

The craniofacial areas, of particular interest in this text, are the nose, the eye, and the ear. The other areas of the face and cranium, eg, the mandible, the lips, and the cheeks, are usually best reconstructed with autogenous tissue.

The nose can be reconstructed with either a laminated forehead flap or a laminated free flap from, for instance, the forearm. The lamination consists of the addition of cartilage grafts for a scaffold for the tip as well as the ala of the nose, adding split-thickness skin grafts for the inside lining of the nose. Usually the forehead flap is preferred, if available, if the donor site defect is acceptable to the patient. This procedure is usually a two- or three-stage surgical procedure. If septal cartilage is available, this can usually be used for support of the nose; otherwise bone or cartilage grafts may need to be used to give the nose proper support and projection. If a nasal reconstruction with autogenous tissue is at all feasible, this is usually my first choice.

Limited defects of the eyelids can usually be reconstructed with autogenous tissue with an excellent esthetic result. If an orbital exenteration has been performed with removal of not only the globe and periorbital fat but also the eyelids, autogenous reconstruction is usually not feasible. These patients are usually best treated with a prosthesis retained by osseointegrated implants.

Autogenous reconstruction of the ear is usually done with the cartilage scaffold covered with either local skin flaps, or a combination of a temporalis fascial flap with a skin graft on top. Even with the best reconstructive techniques, the constructed ear is often bulky and lacks the elasticity of a normal ear. Moreover, the reconstructive procedures are complicated and often fraught with failure. I therefore prefer an osseointegrated ear prosthesis in most cases where the whole ear needs to be reconstructed.

Recent advancements in diagnostic imaging, craniofacial surgery, microsurgery, and tissue expansion have increased the precision as well as the technical armamentarium for autogenous reconstruction of craniomaxillofacial defects. Despite these advances, I usually prefer to reconstruct the missing ear with an osseointegrated prosthesis, which is also often preferable in extensive orbital defects. Nasal defects are reconstructed with autogenous tissue as well as defects in the other areas of the head and neck.

Opportunity for Maxillofacial Prosthetics

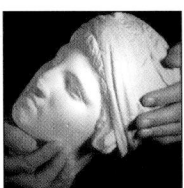

Patrick Henry

The advent of bone-anchored craniofacial prosthetics has expanded the horizons of maxillofacial prosthetic rehabilitation in the past 10 years. Improvements in diagnostic imaging, surgical techniques, and treatment technologies have resulted in higher survival rates and extended longevity for cancer victims. Accordingly, health professionals in this area are increasingly called upon to find solutions for residual cancer defects in patients who hitherto would not have survived. The demands on manpower and resources for such patients can be huge. Because the time frame of extensive osseointegrated-based rehabilitation is long, the maxillofacial prosthodontists or prosthetists inevitably develop a close lifelong relationship with these patients, quite unlike anything seen elsewhere in dentistry and special even compared to most areas of medicine.

While life can be extended by medical science, the quality of that life is another consideration. Furthermore, it is inevitable that eventually that life will pass, and, toward the end, the demands made on the maxillofacial prosthetic therapist may be extreme.

Treatment Opportunities

The complex case involving the middle one-third of the craniofacial skeleton with combined intraoral and extraoral defects represents the greatest challenge. This situation implies loss of speech and masticatory function, and esthetic compromise. The aim of treatment is to give the patient the ability to communicate, masticate, and enjoy a level of social acceptance. Fundamentally, the patient must accept the treatment result in terms of a positive contribution to restoration of lost body parts and self-image. The central issue involved, and the most important goal, is that of communication.

Individuals rendered permanently mute as a result of laryngeal trauma or surgery are likely to better cope with their situation than persons who cannot talk because of extensive loss of palatal, oral, and nasal structure. This latter group of patients becomes deeply frustrated and depressed because the sounds they utter are unintelligible and often interpreted as moronic or alcoholic, especially on the telephone. In the former group, the patient understands that speech is no longer possible, whereas those in the latter group live in desperation and frustration because they can make sounds, but cannot be understood.

The ability to communicate enables the patient to partake of life and to socialize. Even the recluse can communicate via telephone, provided speech can be prosthetically facilitated and the sense of helplessness diminished.

Figure 3-1 illustrates the plight of a woman who was severely injured and disfigured in a motor vehicle accident. After 62 surgical procedures, the patient found her way to our clinic. When asked what her chief problem was, her reply—written on her note pad—was, "I want to be able to communicate."

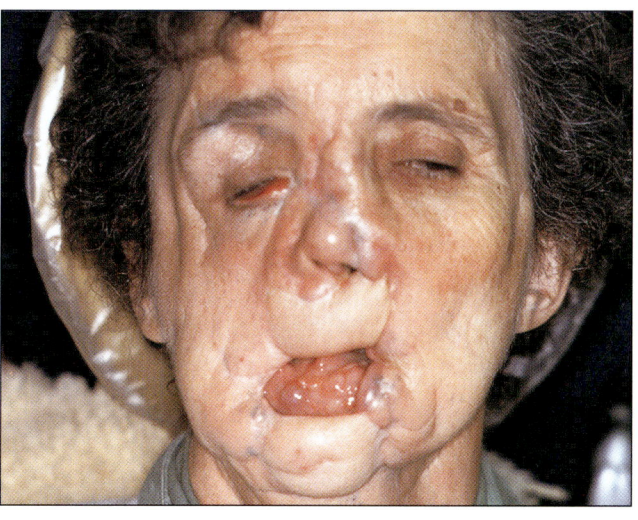

Fig 3-1a This 52-year-old woman was severely injured and disfigured in a motor vehicle accident. Among the extensive intraoral defects were loss of the palate and hemimaxillectomy, hemimandibulectomy, and partial glossectomy.

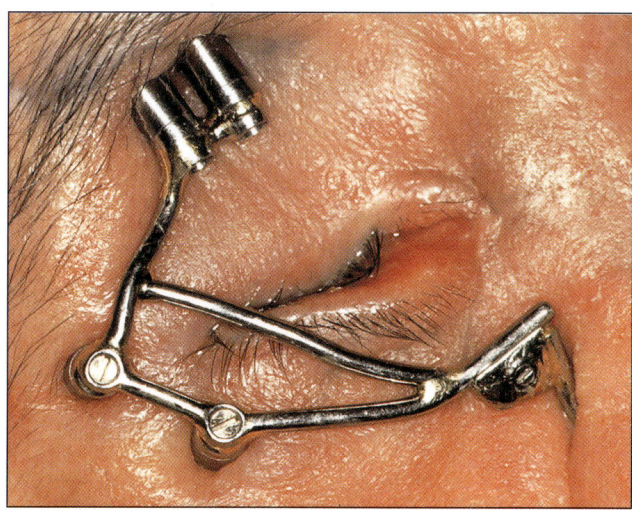

Fig 3-1b After retreatment for intraoral complications, an orbital anchorage system was placed, enabling the placement of an external facial prosthesis and an internal palatal obturator.

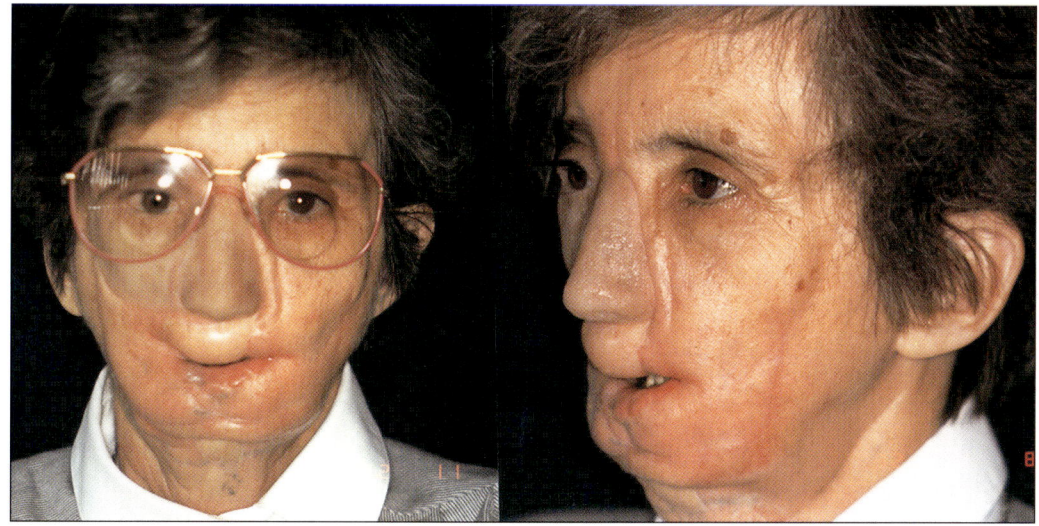

Fig 3-1c The patient with prosthesis in place (two views).

An extensive program of bone-anchored prosthetic rehabilitation was performed, together with intensive speech therapy, enabling the patient to talk on the telephone and in person. However, treatment was not without complications. The palate was initially restored with a bone-anchored segmented overdenture opposing a lower jaw implant bridge, but implant loss in the residual maxillary segment resulted in its demise 1 year later.

Subsequently, the palate was replaced with an obturator using the extended bar of the orbital anchorage system for retention, thus restoring speech and communication for the second time using the principle of flexibility of treatment planning and contingency planning. In the first instance, such cases may be planned to provide excess anchorage potential, where possible, to be prepared for complications. With osseointegrated implants, undertreatment must be avoided. In complex cases, the treatment plan must embrace aspects of long-term maintenance and monitoring and must delineate built-in therapeutic reserve to allow for unforeseen setbacks.

Treatment Limitations

The team approach to treatment gives both the patient and the therapist the best opportunity for good results and optimal management. Even though the principle of team management is well established, it is unfortunately not universal, and may be especially lacking in remote areas. This principle is cardinal in the management of the borderline case of limited prognosis and in the decision-making process of whether or not to treat with bone-anchored prosthetic rehabilitation.

Because early rehabilitation treatment offers psychological advantages to patients, further consideration must be given to the simultaneous resection and conjoint rehabilitation grafting procedure with implants installed at the time of tumor resection. Such procedures are currently limited to experienced teams in major centers. Conversely, the decision to go ahead with extensive placement of implants—dictating an exhaustive prosthetic program in a patient of dubious prognosis—must be carefully rationalized. These difficult decisions are eased by the team approach whereby an oncology board (involving a complete representation of the therapeutic and rehabilitation professional cross-section) can decide what is in the best interest of the patient in light of the fiscal and logistic constraints.

To be avoided is the situation where the prosthetic services department becomes a dumping ground for uninformed patients with poor prognoses, referred from surgical or radiation therapy departments as "hopeless" and "no further treatment indicated."

Patient education, in the form of videotape, with or without the opportunity to talk to successfully treated patients, can be of enormous benefit to cancer patients. In our clinic, such opportunities have had a positive impact in selected circumstances and resulted in the facilitation of the treatment plan with simplification of the logistics.

Recurrence and Terminal Disease

Frequently, strong personal bonds are formed between patients and therapists due to the long treatment regimen and the subsequent lifelong maintenance program. As such, it is likely that the maxillofacial prosthetic profession will face the possibility of having to take on a family-type responsibility where no family exists. This can be put to the test in the face of recurrent or terminal disease. So the ability to work with sick, old, and dying patients is mandatory for maxillofacial professionals.

The patient's anger in the early stages of the dying process is not to be interpreted personally by the therapist and care must be taken not to develop an avoidance pattern in response to hostile behavior. Avoidance may be counterproductive in relation to the tissue and prosthesis maintenance needs and management in later stages. Although treatment encounters may be potentially uncomfortable or painful for the maxillofacial professional, understanding and respect for the patient are required at this time. In some cases, the professional will be targeted as incapable and possibly even blamed for the recurrent disease. Generally, this attitude will soften as the patient moves into later stages.

Palliative care units and hospice facilities have progressed considerably in recent years in terms of environment, philosophy, and standard of care. Many have 24-hour care and, accordingly, multiple staff changes. Attendant staff require instruction in implant hygiene, tissue health, and maintenance and care of the prosthesis as the patient becomes increasingly incapable or disinterested in self-care. Bone-anchored prostheses are still a source of intense interest for palliative care staff, most of whom know little of the science or background for this recently developed modality. Unfortunately, guidelines for care following late or repetitive radiation therapy or chemotherapy are still uncertain, and careful observation and evaluation are required of the maxillofacial prosthodontist at palliative follow-up.

Patient Response to Rehabilitation

One of the early pioneer patients is seen in Figure 3-2 shortly after transfer to a palliative care unit 10 years after implant installation. This patient was treated for total maxillectomy and mid-third facial resection with a bone-anchored maxillary overdenture, with the bone-anchorage system also providing retention for the facial camouflage prosthesis. The treatment transformed his life from that of a recluse into one of virtual normalcy.

The vast majority of patients believe their treatment was instrumental in giving them quality of life after life itself was almost lost. This positive response has encouraged those in the field to promote and expand the bone-anchored application. Today we are only beginning to see the possibilities. Tomorrow many more patients will have the opportunity of further improved quality of life through bone-anchored prosthetic techniques.

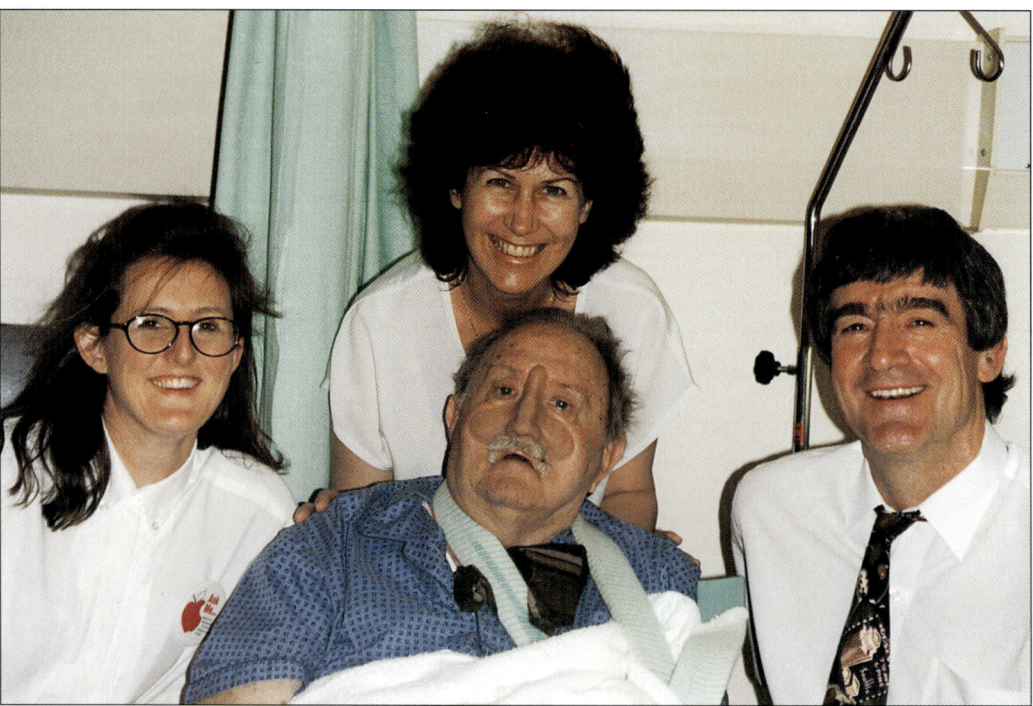

Fig 3-2 Early pioneer patient 10 years after implant placement with members of the Perth osseointegration team. He described his treatment as having given him an additional 10 years enjoyment of life.

Anaplastological Technique for Facial Defects

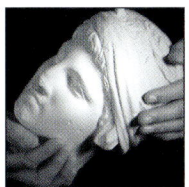

Kerstin Bergström

Before a patient undergoes surgery, he or she should be seen by the prosthetic rehabilitation team so that information about the ongoing and future treatment plans can be shared. At that time, an impression and photographs of the area can be taken, facilitating the prosthetic work. If the anaplastologist can be in the operating theater and discuss the size, depth, and surface contour of the defect to be created with the surgeon, this will optimize the design of the subsequent prosthesis.

When placing craniofacial implants, it is important that the surgeon discusses the position and direction of the fixtures with the anaplastologist to achieve a good final result (Fig 4-1) and to facilitate cleaning around the abutment.

For an auricular prosthesis, for instance, two implants are normally sufficient for satisfactory retention, and the ideal position is approximately 20 mm from the center of the ear canal opening. On the right side the positions are at eight o'clock and eleven o'clock. On the left side, the corresponding positions are at four o'clock and one o'clock (Fig 4-2).

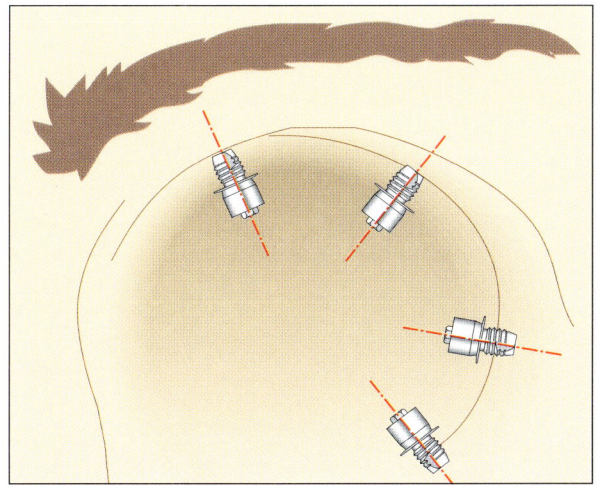

Fig 4-1

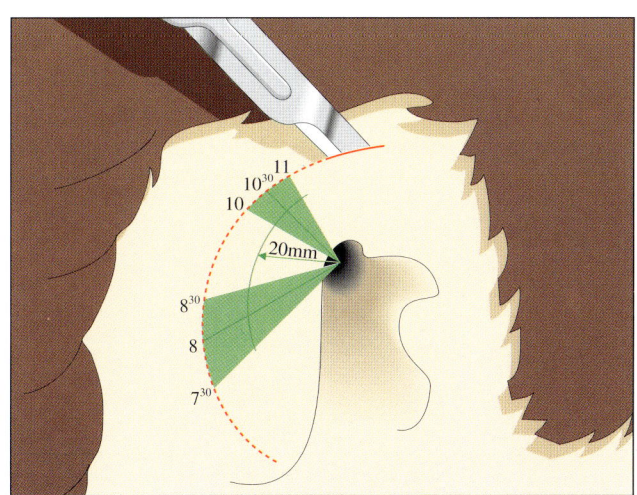

Fig 4-2

The distance between the fixtures should be at least 15 mm if possible, depending on the anatomic situation. For an orbital prosthesis, it is not only the position, but also the direction and number of implants that should be considered. If possible, it is more favorable to have more than two fixtures placed both in the upper and lower orbital rims.

PREPROSTHETIC PLANNING

When planning the prosthesis fabrication, several types of retention can be used, depending on several factors such as: size, depth, and location of the defect; position and number of implants; loading situation; mobility of the surrounding tissue; and age and ability of the patient.

TYPES OF RETENTION

Bar Construction and Retentive Clips
A bar construction is a wire soldered to gold cylinders and mounted onto the abutments by gold screws. Such a construction provides a good load distribution on the implants. Retentive clips are placed on the inner aspect of the acrylic plate, providing a rigid and secure position for the prosthesis. For auricular prostheses and for large orbital prostheses where implants have been placed in the upper orbital rim, this kind of retention is recommended (Fig 4-3).

Individual Magnets
The individual retention system consists of a magnet cap that is threaded onto the abutment and a magnet placed into the fitting side of the prosthesis. In an orbital defect with implants in the upper and lower orbital rim, the individual magnet system is recommended. It is especially recommended when there is a shallow defect with insufficient space for a bar-and-clip construction. For the patient, it is very easy to put on and take off the prosthesis and to properly clean around the abutments (Fig 4-4).

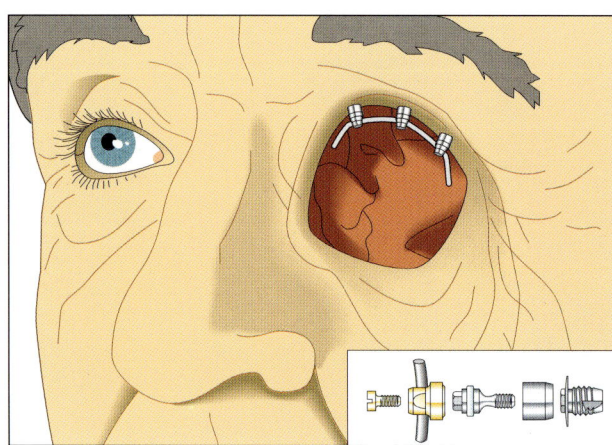

Fig 4-3

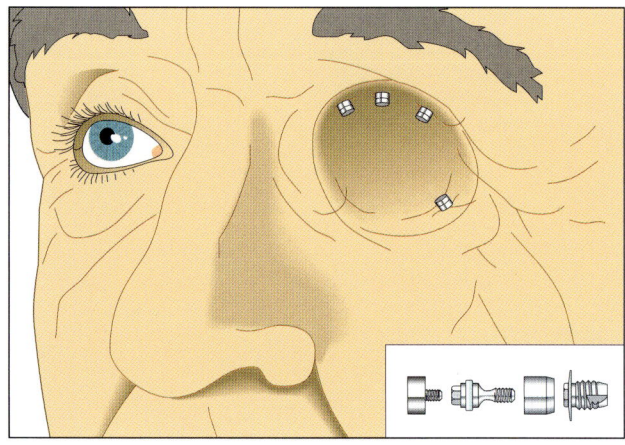

Fig 4-4

Ball Attachments
When there is a shallow defect, the ball attachments are one option of retention because they take little space behind the prosthesis. Three implants creating a tripod are imperative to provide satisfactory retention and stability (Fig 4-5). In addition to the systems mentioned, there are others that can be used depending on the individual situation.[1]

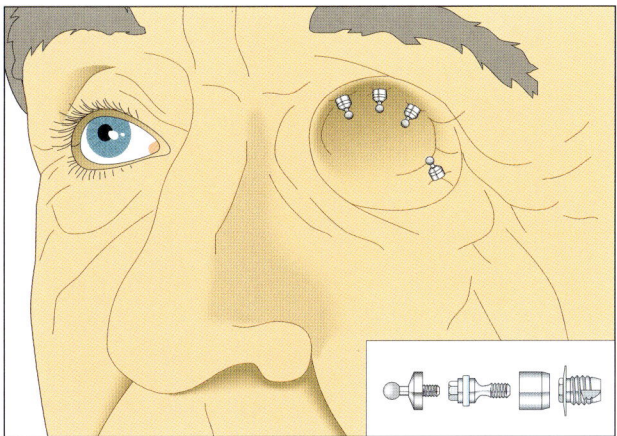

Fig 4-5

Fabrication of an Auricular Prosthesis

When the wound has healed sufficiently, normally 3 to 4 weeks after abutment placement (for a two-stage procedure), it is possible to start the fabrication of the prosthesis (Fig 4-6).

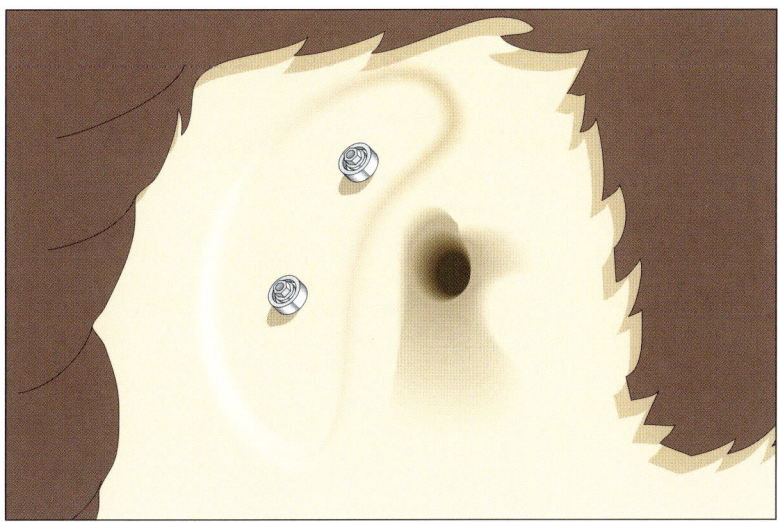

Fig 4-6

Impression

The first step is to make a working model in plaster, reproducing detailed anatomic information of the defect area, and a precise position of the abutments. Impression copings with long guide pins are attached to the percutaneous abutments. A low-viscosity alginate mixture is used to make the impression, and a thin layer is applied around the copings and over the entire area required for making the prosthesis. It is important not to cover the impression copings with alginate. Pieces of gauze are then placed on the surface of the alginate. When the alginate has set, the top of the box is filled with impression plaster. This secures the impression copings in position and stabilizes the alginate impression material. It is important not to cover the guide pins with impression plaster (Fig 4-7).

When the plaster has set, the guide pins are unscrewed and the impression is removed. Abutment replicas are then attached to the impression copings, and the impression is cast in dental stone (Fig 4-8).

When the impression material is separated from the cast, an exact working model of the patient's defect area will be created with the abutment replicas in exactly the same position, direction, and height as the skin-penetrating abutments (Fig 4-9). An impression of the opposite ear is taken to facilitate the sculpturing of the prosthesis (Fig 4-10).

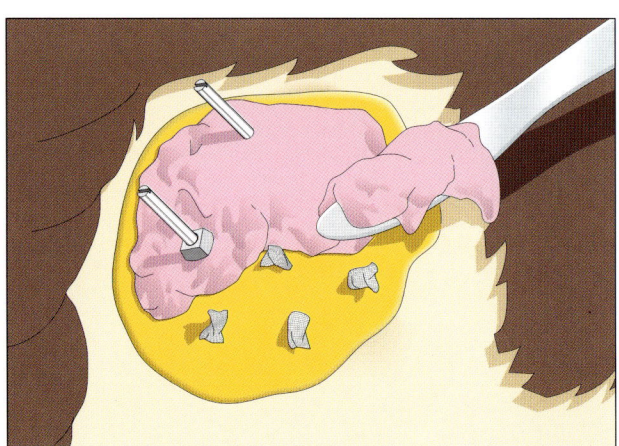

Fig 4-7

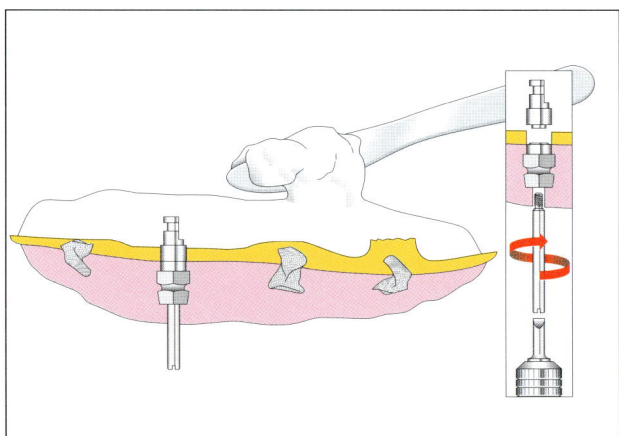

Fig 4-8

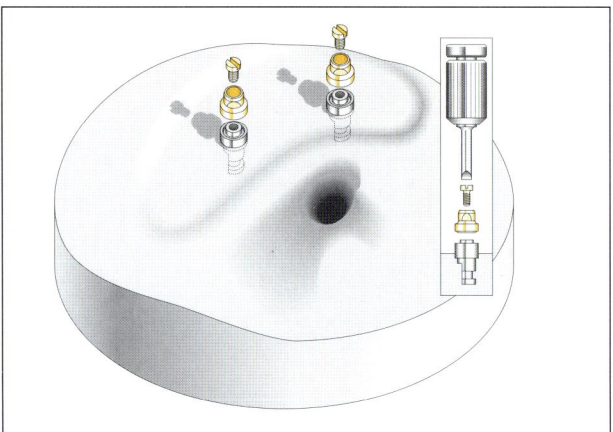

Fig 4-9

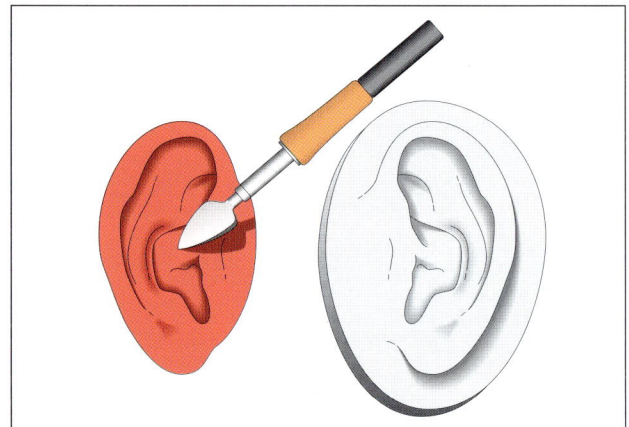

Fig 4-10

Framework

The design of the framework is determined, and a drawing of the shape is made. It is desirable to have the bar under the anti-helix part of the ear.

The gold cylinders are placed on the abutment replicas of the working model, and a 2-mm gold bar is attached to the gold cylinders with sticky wax or acrylic (Fig 4-11). The bar should not extend more than 8 to 10 mm beyond the abutment to reduce bending movement to the fixtures (Fig 4-12).

The bar is removed from the model and invested for soldering. After soldering, the bar is carefully checked on the working cast and on the patient for a passive fit.

Retention clips are then positioned on the bar, and an acrylic plate is made. The acrylic resin plate is tried on the patient to verify fit and contours.

The wax ear is positioned onto the acrylic plate on the patient to identify the correct orientation (Fig 4-13). A 2-mm space is left between the skin and acrylic plate at the back of the prosthesis, allowing air access to skin to prevent irritation due to moisture accumulation.[2]

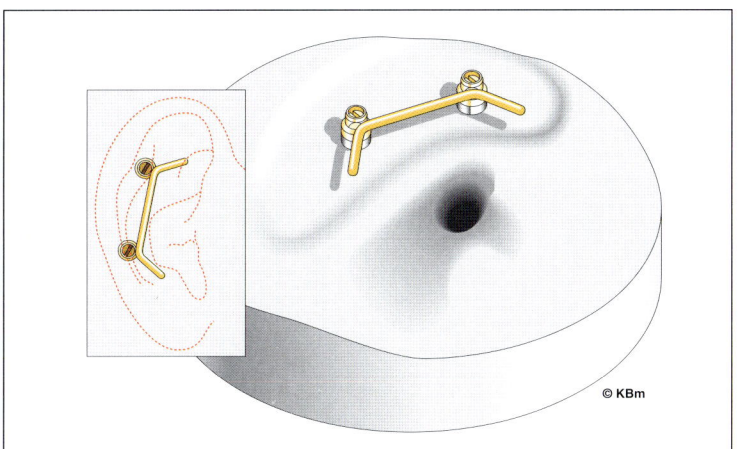

Fig 4-11

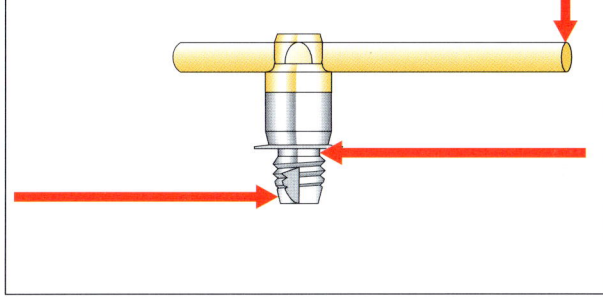

Fig 4-12

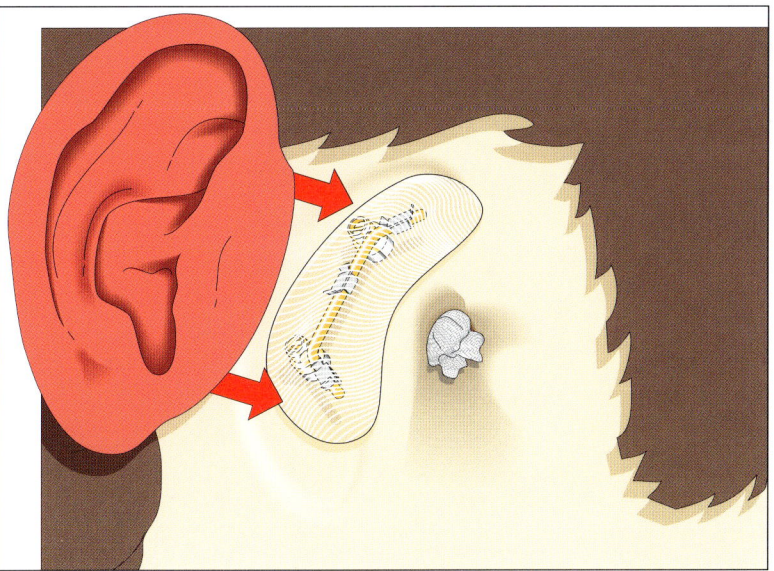

Fig 4-13

When the wax ear model and the acrylic plate have an optimal fit (Fig 4-14), the ear and bar are embedded in a mold of plaster stone, which consists of three parts (Fig 4-15).

The wax is then removed with boiling water (Fig 4-16), and before the mold is packed with silicone, the acrylic plate must be prepared in the following way to achieve strong bonding: 1) the surface is roughened with a stone; 2) the external surface is cleaned with acetone; and 3) the primer is applied in two thin layers and allowed to dry.

The silicone is mixed with colors to match the different skin shades of the patient (Fig 4-17). When the silicone has polymerized, the prosthesis is carefully removed from the mold and trimmed. Extrinsic tinting is applied if necessary. The prosthesis is delivered to the patient with instructions for care of the skin around the abutments and care of the prosthesis (Fig 4-18).

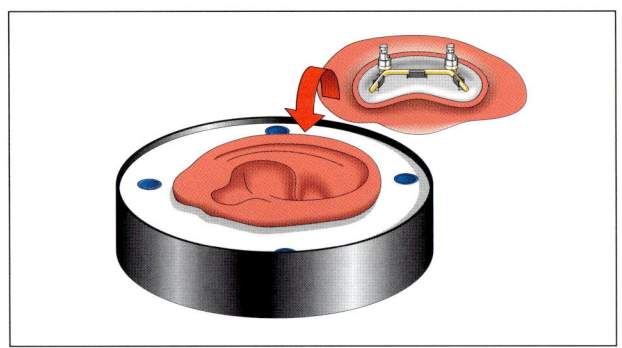

Fig 4-14

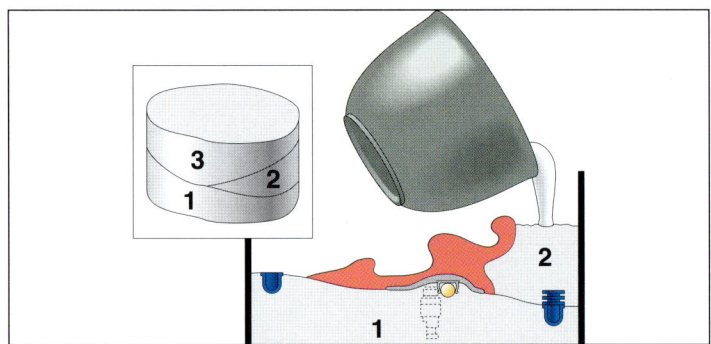

Fig 4-15

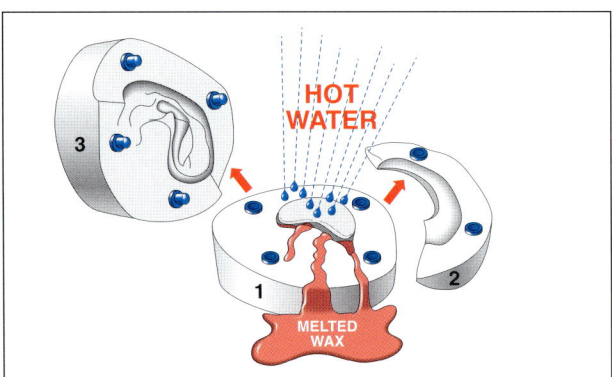

Fig 4-16

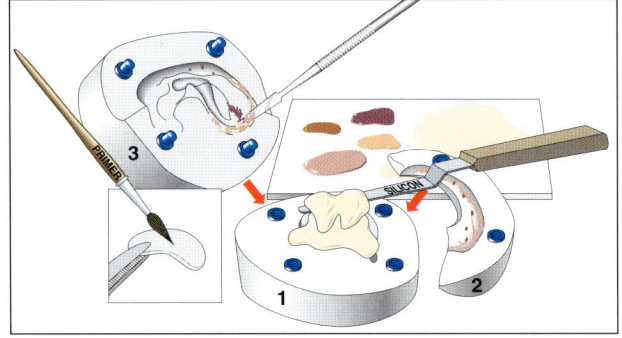

Fig 4-17

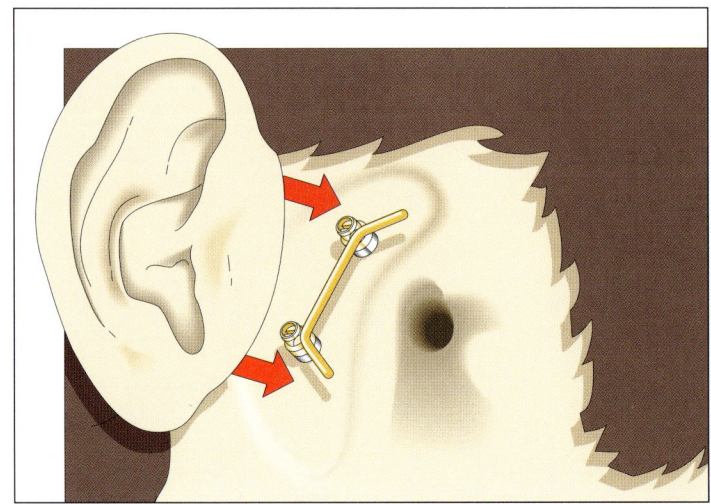

Fig 4-18

Fabrication of an Orbital Prosthesis

Although technically similar to fabrication of an auricular prosthesis, fabrication of an orbital prosthesis is more complex and requires more from the rehabilitating team.

Take the following case: A patient has had three implants placed in the supraorbital rim. A bar with clips is selected as the most appropriate retention for the prosthesis, since there are implants only in the upper orbital rim (Fig 4-19). If fixtures have been placed in both upper and lower orbital rims, there is generally more choice in the method of retention eg, individual magnets or ball attachments.

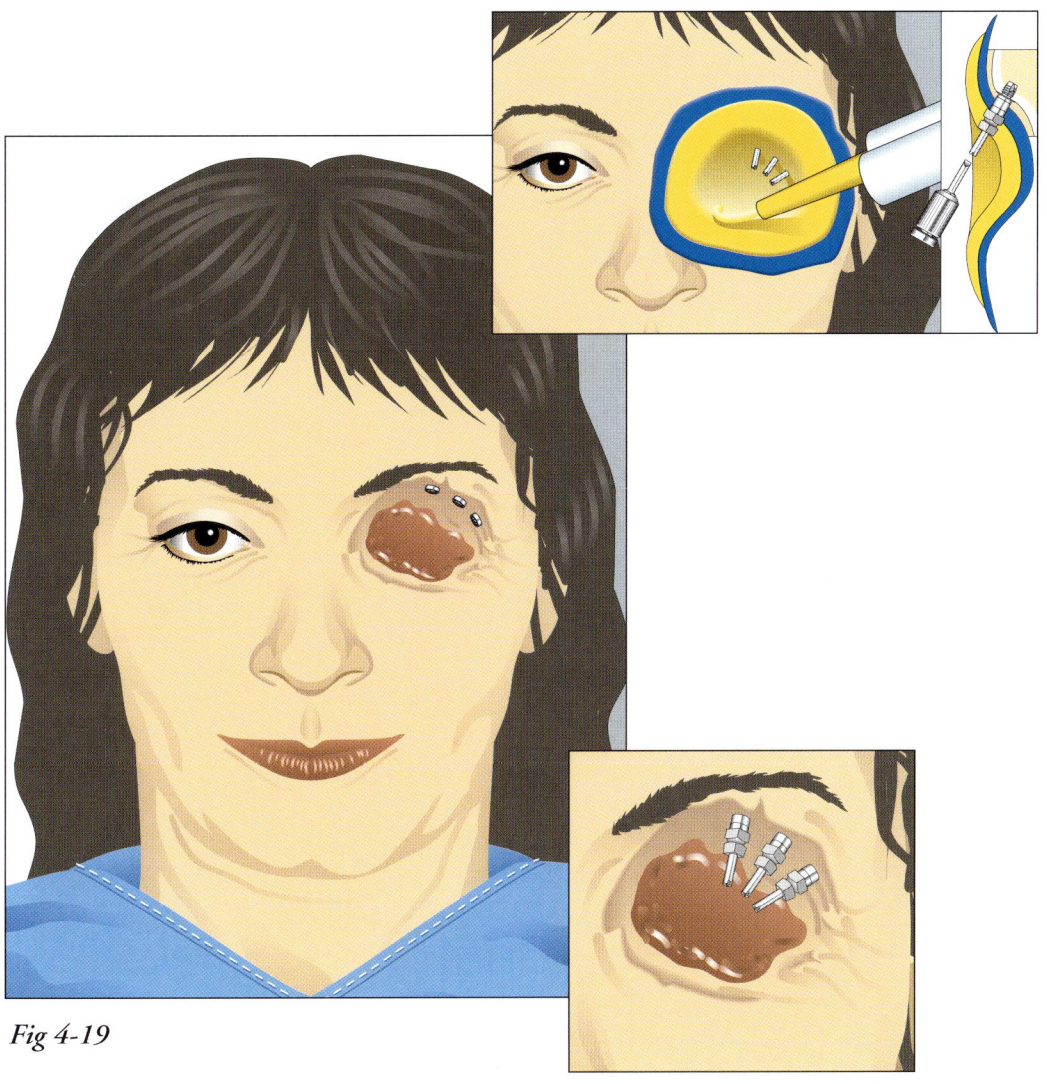

Fig 4-19

POSITIONING OF THE ARTIFICIAL EYE

The bar and acrylic plate are placed on the patient, and the artificial eye is positioned on the acrylic plate at an approximate position with a piece of soft wax. Both the height and depth of the eye must be measured using the other eye as a guide. The exact distance from the midline of the face is also important. The final position of the eye has to be determined with care and with the patient in both a sitting and standing position, because the appearance differs. Correct positioning of the eye in all three planes is of utmost importance for the final result of the orbital prosthesis (Fig 4-20).

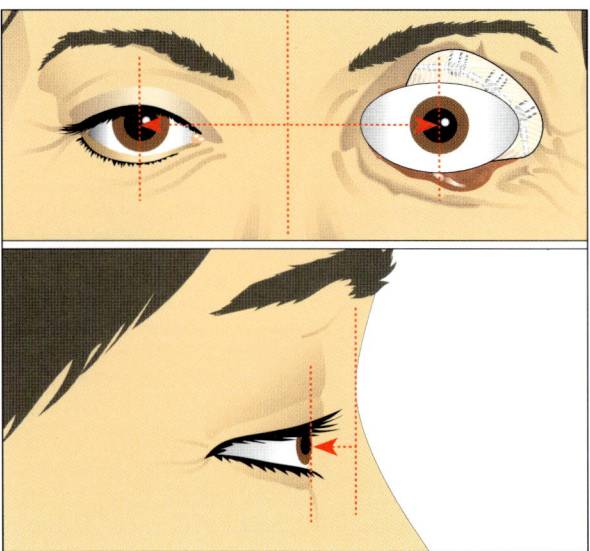

Fig 4-20

SCULPTURING

The sculpturing of the wax prosthesis is made on both the master cast and on the patient. To achieve a lifelike orbital restoration, it is important to pay attention to details. Also, the edge of the wax prosthesis has to be made extremely thin to achieve an invisible junction between the artificial material and the skin. It is important to find the most favorable extension of the prosthesis considering the size and contour of the defect.

Mold Fabrication

A two-piece plaster mold is made and created to be used several times in the future for remakes or spare prostheses. An acrylic locating key is attached to the artificial eye to be retained in the second part of the mold (Fig 4-21). The plaster is smoothed with sandpaper, and a thin film of separating agent is applied on the plaster. The second part of the mold is poured. Once separated and cleaned, the two-part mold is left with the acrylic plate and artificial eye in place.

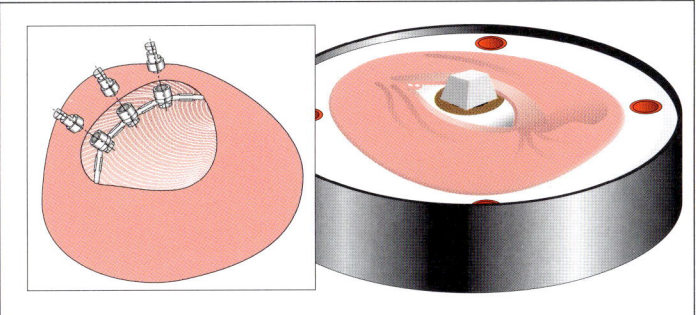

Fig 4-21

Silicone Processing

A primary concern is to assure a chemical bond between the acrylic plate and the silicone.

Esthetics are optimized by creating as much staining through intrinsic color as possible. Silicone is packed in the mold in matched segments (Fig 4-22), and the mold is closed for processing.

When the vulcanization is completed, the mold is opened, and the prosthesis margins are trimmed.

Eyelashes are inserted in the silicone with a special tool (Fig 4-23). The prosthesis is now tried on the patient, and if necessary, final extrinsic color adjustments can be made.[3]

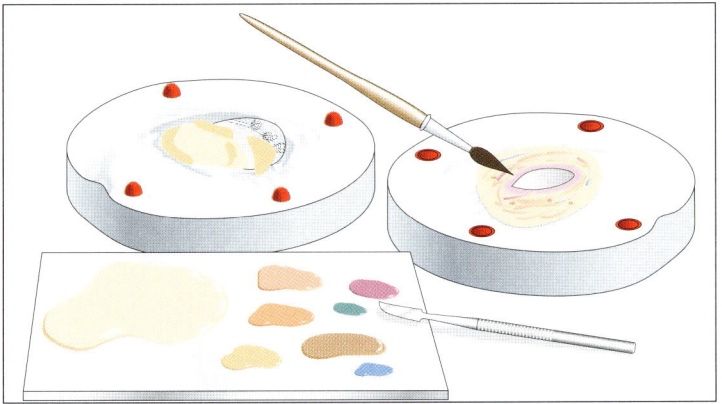

Fig 4-22

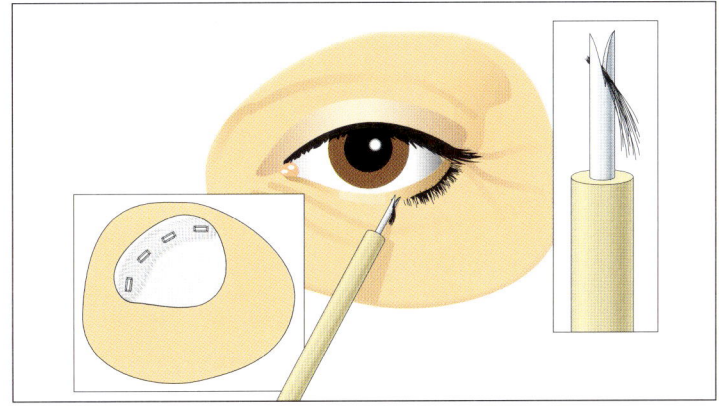

Fig 4-23

REFERENCES

1. Bergström K. Prosthetic procedures for orbital defects: Technique and case study. J Facial Somato Prosthetics 1996; 2(1):27–35.
2. Tjellström A, Jansson K, Brånemark P-I. Craniofacial defects. In: Worthington P, Brånemark P-I (eds.) Advanced Osseointegration Surgery. Applications in the Maxillofacial Region. Chicago: Quintessence, 1992: 293–312.
3. Tjellström A, Granström G, Bergström K. Osseointegrated implants for craniofacial prostheses. In: Weber R, Miller MJ, Goepfert H (eds). Basal and Squamous Cell Skin Cancers of the Head and Neck. Baltimore: Williams & Wilkins, 1996:313–330.

Impaired Function of the Temporomandibular Joint in Oncology Patients

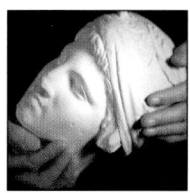

Ragnar Adell

A PATIENT WHO NOT ONLY SUFFERS from a malignancy in the oral maxillofacial region but *also* sustains a restricted function in one or both temporomandibular joints (TMJs) is subject to a most critical situation. The inability to open one's mouth causes nutritional problems and an increased risk of dental and periodontal diseases due to impaired ability to perform adequate oral hygiene. Moreover, such diseases may prove difficult to treat due to lack of access. For most patients, however, the greatest problems of a restricted mouth opening are the psychosocial implications and the realistic fear of not being able to maintain an adequate airway in an emergency situation.

Etiology

Impaired TMJ function in oncology patients is generally due to one or more of the following problems. Ablative surgery in the face and neck region can give rise to scar tissue contractions, which restrict mandibular movements.[1] Irradiation of the chewing muscles causes muscle fibrosis. The TMJ has to be partially or totally ablated when a tumor is located in the joint area. TMJ resection may also turn out to be necessary when an adjacent malignancy, such as in the mandibular ramus or the parotid gland, has to be removed. Its radical excision may then require that the condyle also has to be exarticulated.

Treatment Modalities

The skull base, the TMJ region, the mandibular ramus, and the zygomatic and infrazygomatic regions should all be well delineated with computed tomographic (CT) scans or magnetic resonance imaging (MRI) before any treatment is instituted.

Two principles are important for good treatment results relating to restricted TMJ function. One is effective lifelong physiotherapy, which should be applied in every case, irrespective of additional treatment options. A variety of approaches may be taken, from finger-assisted exercises to hightech.[2] It is important to start a mandibular-opening maintenance program as soon as a restriction in opening capacity is diagnosed, and to maintain it daily and forever. Severe difficulties with physiotherapy exercises may, however, arise if an irradiated and, maybe, partially resected, mandible is prone to pathologic fractures. Apart from physiotherapy, forced manipulation under general anesthesia can be tried. Treatment with hyperbaric oxygen has also been suggested (D. Zeitler, personal communication, 1988).

The second principle is that of radical and aggressive surgery[3] when physiotherapy alone does not help. Scar tissue contraction from previous surgery is treated by excision and the addition of well-vascularized fresh tissue[4,5] always followed by early, aggressive, and continuous physiotherapy.

When surgery is indicated, the choice of method primarily depends on whether or not the intracapsular TMJ components remain intact. If the intra-articular parts do not show any pathological changes in the preoperative CT or MRI studies, a most thorough stripping of the stylomandibular tendon and all muscular attachments (temporalis, masseter, and pterygoids) from the mandibular ramus through preauricular, submandibular, and/or intraoral approaches may be sufficient. In this approach, the muscles are not sutured back but left to reinsert at a more functional level. The release of the temporalis attachment is effectively performed by a coronoidectomy. In every long-standing case of mandibular hypomobility, there is a risk of disuse atrophy or muscle fibrosis on the contralateral side as well. The outcome of stripping muscle and tendon attachments on the affected side only should always be checked intraoperatively by forced manipulation.

In most cases, it will be found that a similar procedure is also needed on the contralateral side to achieve an optimal interincisal opening (defined as more than 35 mm[3]). Consequently, the patient must be informed preoperatively about the possibility of a bilateral approach. If sufficient mouth opening is not achieved by these means, the intracapsular joint components should be examined for possible intra-articular reasons for the trismus and treated accordingly.

If the intra-articular components are pathologically involved, TMJ replacement may be necessary (Figs 5-1 to 5-3). All of the above tendon and muscle stripping must also be performed simultaneously. In the case, for example, of a benign tumor in the condylar head or mandibular ramus, a costochondral graft with about a 1-mm chondral part and a perichondrium-periosteal collar will generally provide an excellent substitute.[6] The graft is taken from the fifth or sixth rib of the opposing side. The posterior-lateral surface of the mandibular ramus and the corresponding part of the graft are well decorticated and the transplant is fixed by two bone screws or a miniplate. Details of the costochondral grafting techniques and the composition of the graft have been discussed by Svensson et al.[7] This method also offers favorable prospects for growing individuals. Its clinical application in a benign tumor case was recently described.[8]

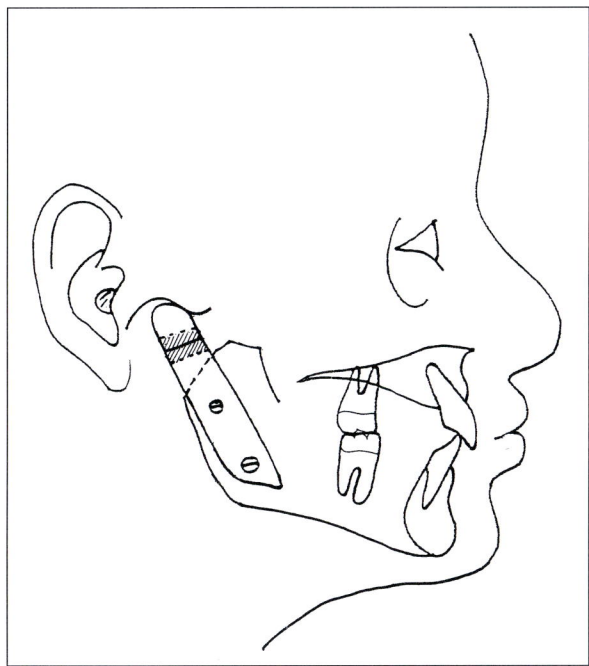

Fig 5-1 *Schematic illustration of a costochondral graft with a perichondrium-periosteal collar to replace a resected mandibular condyle. The graft is fixed with two osteosynthesis screws to the lateral surface of the ramus of the mandible.*

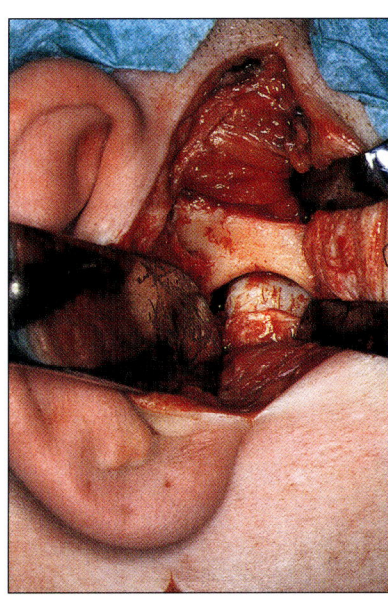

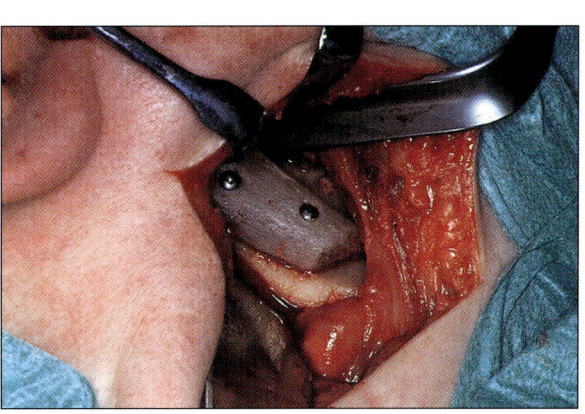

Fig 5-2a and b Corresponding clinical views in the preauricular area (a) and from a submandibular view (b).

In the case of a TMJ or ramus malignancy, immediate reconstruction is usually not recommended.[9] An excellent intermediate or possibly permanent reconstruction is then offered by the THORP system or its successor, the Locking Screw Mandibular Plating System with an alloplastic condylar head.[10,11]

For the more extensive permanent reconstructions of the mandibular body, ramus, neck and condyle, alternative approaches may include various kinds of cribs filled with autologous Particulate Bone Cancellous Marrow, PBCM bone,[1] preformed bone grafts with incorporated implants for attachment and support,[12] or preferably microsurgically anastomosed grafts.[13–15]

POSTOPERATIVE REGIMEN

The early and aggressive postoperative physiotherapy regimen can not be overemphasized. After a short period of maxillomandibular fixation, patients are started on a soft diet and gradually more demanding jaw opening exercises, possibly using specially designed jaw exercising machines.[2]

References

1. Marx RE, Sunders TR. Reconstruction and rehabilitation of cancer patients. In: Fonseca RJ, Davis WH (eds). Reconstructive Pre-prosthetic Oral Maxillofacial Surgery. Philadelphia: WB Saunders, 1986.
2. Buchbinder D, Currivan RB, Kaplan AJ, Urken ML. Mobilisation regimens for the prevention of jaw hypomobility in the radiated patient: A comparison of three techniques. J Oral Maxillofac Surg 1993;51:863–867.
3. Kaban LB, Perrot DH, Fischer K. A protocol for management of temporomandibular joint ankylosis. J Oral Maxillofac Surg 1990;48:1145–1151.
4. Chen Z, Chen C. Correction of extra-capsular temporo-mandibular joint ankylosis with a cervical subcutaneous pedicle flap. Plast Reconstr Surg 1990;86:138–141.
5. Hill AJ. Release of mandibular ankylosis due to gross tissue loss in the cheek. Int J Oral Surg 1978;7:369–373.
6. Obeid G, Guttenberg SA, Connole PW. Costochondral grafting in condylar replacement and mandibular reconstruction. J Oral Maxillofac Surg 1988;46:177–182.
7. Svensson B, Feldmann G, Rindler N. Early surgical-orthodontic treatment of mandibular hypoplasia in juvenile chronic arthritis. J Craniomaxillofac Surg 1993;21:67–75.
8. Svensson B, Isacsson G. Benign osteoblastoma associated with an aneurysmal bone cyst of the mandibular ramus and condyle. Oral Surg Oral Med Oral Pathol 1993;76:433–436.
9. Lindqvist C, Söderholm A-L, Laine P, Paatsama J. Rigid reconstruction plates for immediate reconstruction following mandibular resection for malignant tumours. J Oral Maxillofac Surg 1992;50:1158–1163.
10. Vuillemin T, Raveh J, Sutter F. Mandibular reconstruction with the THORP condylar prosthesis after hemi-mandibelectomy. J Craniomaxillofac Surg 1989;17:78–87.
11. Hellem S, Olofsson J. Titanium-coated hollow screw and reconstruction plate system THORP in mandibular reconstruction. J Craniomaxillofac Surg 1988;16:173–183.
12. Brånemark P-I, Lindström J, Hallén O, Breine U, Jeppson PH, Öhman A. Reconstruction of the defective mandible. Scand J Dent Plast Reconstr Surg 1975;9:116–128.
13. Schmelzeisen R, Rhan BA, Brennwald J. Fixation of vascularized bone grafts. J Craniomaxillofac Surg 1993;21:113–119.
14. Urken ML. Composite free flaps in oromandibular reconstruction; review of the literature. Arch Otolaryngol Head Neck Surg 1991;117:724–732.
15. Urken ML, Weinberg H, Vickery C, Buchbinder D, Lawson W, Biller HF. Oromandibular reconstruction using microvascular composite free flaps: report of 71 cases and a new classification scheme for bony, soft-tissue and neurologic defects. Arch Otolaryngol Head Neck Surg 1991;117:733–744.

Hyperbaric Oxygen Treatment of Former Cancer Patients to Support Osseointegration

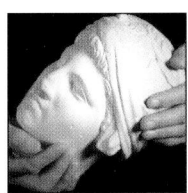

Gösta Granström

Since the introduction of extraoral osseointegrated implants in 1977, an increasing number of patients have been treated with this modality. In our department, in 17 years, 241 patients have had implants placed for rehabilitation with extraoral prostheses, including: 158 ear prostheses, 48 orbit prostheses, 15 midface or nasal prostheses, and 20 maxillary or mandibular reconstructions. Of the total, 178 patients were rehabilitated after tumor surgery, and of these patients 45 were irradiated before implant surgery.

Placing titanium implants in irradiated bone was originally contraindicated, and some clinics today still take a very conservative attitude toward treating such patients. We have 13 years' follow-up of irradiated patients treated in our clinic,[1] and statistics show an increased loss of implants in these patients compared to nonirradiated patients. The highest implant losses were observed during the first 3 years after implant surgery, after which time fewer implants were lost, but implant losses continued throughout the 13 years recorded.

Implants are lost in two ways: either the fixtures are found at the second stage to not have integrated or the patients lose implants, generally without considerable trauma. After such an event, the implant site has usually healed within 3 to 4 weeks without causing any severe tissue reactions such as continuous drainage, fistulation, or bone necrosis. To be able to wear a prosthesis, the patient has generally been supplied with new implants.

In total over the period, implants losses were 37% in irradiated patients, with significant differences between the various facial bones. The highest implant losses were seen in the supraorbital rim, 55%; followed by lateral orbital rim, 40%; lower jaw, 33%; upper jaw, 14%; and mastoid, 9%.

Hyperbaric Oxygen Treatment

To improve implant integration and implant survival rate and to reduce the risk of osteoradionecrosis and other surgical complications, we have performed implant surgery with HBO as a supplement in all radiated patients for the past 6 years. The reason for this treatment is growing understanding of basic biologic reactions in the irradiated tissue and that, to some extent, these effects can be counteracted by HBO.[2]

The protocol has been to pretreat patients with the equivalent of 20 oxygen dives at 2.5 times absolute atmospheric pressure, 90 minutes daily, followed by first-stage implant surgery and immediate postoperative treatment with another 10 oxygen dives.

Second-stage surgery is performed 6 to 8 months after first-stage surgery without any additional HBO.[3] Using this regimen, we have improved implant survival significantly. Six years of follow-up show that after the first year of implant surgery, only one implant has been lost, the difference between non-HBO and HBO groups being significant ($P<0.001$) after this time. By treating the irradiated patients with supplementary HBO, implant losses are reduced to levels similar to those in nonirradiated patients.

Timing of Reconstruction

The optimal time to rehabilitate a tumor patient with osseointegrated implants is not yet established. From the patient's point of view, immediate rehabilitation is desired, but a time lapse of 1 to 3 years after tumor surgery is recommended for the detection of possible secondary tumors. With respect to the radiobiologic considerations, the optimal time for implant surgery would be in the interval between the abatement of post–radiation therapy acute tissue reactions and the establishment of the healing phase; ie, 2 to 4 months after radiation. To reduce the risk of severe tissue reactions due to surgical trauma in the irradiated tissue, 6 months to 1½ years after irradiation would be preferable.[4]

When extraoral implants were first being placed, there was a group of patients with a great need for implant-based rehabilitation who had undergone tumor treatment many years previously. In recent years, however, tumor patients have had implants inserted soon after tumor surgery. Today we supply most patients with implants at the time of surgery. The advantage of this approach is that rehabilitation with the bone-anchored implant system is immediately planned. Using an optimal time-record protocol, this means that the patient can be supplied with the bone-anchored prosthesis as early as 8 weeks after tumor resection. Any tumor recurrence can easily be detected as the tumor cavity is left open for inspection. Because implant surgery has been specially modified to be nontraumatic for tissue, the risk of developing osteoradionecrosis is minimized.

References

1. Granström G, Tjellström A, Brånemark P-I, Fornander J. Bone-anchored reconstruction of the irradiated head and neck cancer patient. Otolaryngol Head Neck Surg 1993;108:334–343.
2. Granström G, Jacobsson M, Tjellström A. Titanium implants in irradiated tissue: Benefits from hyperbaric oxygen. Int J Oral Maxillofac Implants 1992;7:15–25.
3. Granström G. The use of hyperbaric oxygen to prevent implant loss in the irradiated patient. In: Worthington P, Brånemark P-I (eds): Advanced Osseointegration Surgery. Chicago: Quintessence, 1992:336–345.
4. Marx RE, Johnson RP. Studies in the radiobiology of ORN and their clinical significance. Oral Surg Oral Med Oral Pathol 1987;64:379–390.

7

Psychological Considerations in the Treatment of Patients with Cancer

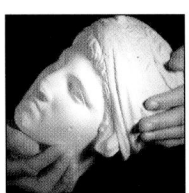

Stig Blomberg

For a patient with cancer, diagnosis and confirmation of a malignancy in the craniofacial region is likely to mean a profound psychological crisis. The patient's capacity to adapt and maintain a psychological balance, through as satisfactory a resolution of the crisis as possible, is crucial for the subsequent surgical treatment.

The criteria for profound psychological vulnerability, which can hinder or contraindicate rehabilitation in complicated cases, have been established previously as: psychotic illness, previous or existing addiction (alcohol, drugs, etc), and pronounced personality disturbance, such as strongly hysterical or narcissistic personality traits.

Teamwork, including a clinical psychologist or psychiatrist who has a thorough knowledge of the field, is of great value. A patient's psychological distress can be eased and adaptation facilitated by a crisis-focused intervention. This can also reduce the emotional strain on the surgeon responsible for the treatment during the long follow-up regimen that is frequently required.

It is the surgeon's responsibility to decide conclusively whether or not to perform the treatment. It is also the surgeon who, in the future, will face the patient's reactions—fear and anxiety, regressive behavior and attitudes, and difficult periods that may end in projective acting out and aggression.

This transference reaction (from the patient to the surgeon) and countertransference (the doctor's response to the patient's reaction) takes place partly in an unconscious way and thus is often not actively recognized. In certain difficult cases, these reactions can so complicate treatment that the entire course of rehabilitation is jeopardized.

Examples of such behavior can be *projective defense*, where the patient cannot accept the existence of a malign illness that cannot be changed despite the amount of professional treatment that is carried out. If the treatment is of long duration, such reactions can be mitigated if the patient's relatives can be supportive during the crisis. Unfortunately, the treatment can also be put at risk if relatives react with denial and projection instead of accepting the situation and managing themselves to integrate the trauma.

If signs of such a reaction are noticed at preoperative assessment sessions or during the early stages of treatment, psychotherapy should be initiated; otherwise, the whole treatment plan is at risk. In such cases, the situation gives rise to inadequate crisis resolution, repression, and denial of the illness/trauma and projection instead of integration and adaptation through the acceptance of the illness and its consequences. This reaction can create emotional stress for the treatment team, including the surgeon. A conscious therapeutic attitude and an understanding of the patient's reaction background can reduce this risk. Factors promoting such a therapeutic attitude are part of a supportive psychotherapy.

1. Professional competence
2. Empathy
3. Continuity (the same surgeon takes responsibility throughout)
4. *Containing function*: treatment personnel tolerate the patient's anxiety and are capable of taking care of the patient's fear
5. *Chaos structuring*: ie, the patient can frequently verbalize anxieties about treatment and the progress of the disease, and get a professional, yet empathetic, response

Through this approach, one can maintain positive transference and the surgeon can be seen as and remain a "good object."

The emotional stress on the treatment surgeon can be reduced through a raised awareness of his or her own reactions. This means watching for any tendency to omnipotence. ("Doctor, you are the only physician who understands me/you are the only one who can cure me.") An overly strong emotional and empathetic commitment or early promise given about long-term treatment can hinder the surgeon's freedom of treatment options and lead to a display of unconscious guilt feelings.

Thus it is important to consider the essential balance in the therapeutic relationship between doctor and patient: accept—set limits; help—make demands; passive observation—active decision; closeness and understanding—distance and overview; objective and professional—human and empathetic.

Emotional stress release can also occur through discussions within the treatment team and consultation with outside colleagues. Most important is one's own clinical experience, maturity, and philosophy of life as a basis for professional work and responsibility.

Facial Reconstruction Following Cancer Treatment: A Case Study

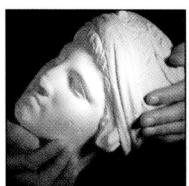

Elaine Williams

New facial tumor cases in Sweden requiring maxillectomy total around 120 per year. In general, it is expected that any radical life-saving tumor-removal surgery will frequently result in severe facial damage.

Survival rates for facial tumors are also unpredictable, as cancers that invade the bone and blood systems tend to be aggressive with local growth or secondary tumors as real risks. This case of a 58-year-old Swedish woman highlights the entire range of treatment dilemmas that can face the rehabilitation team.

During the 11 years that this patient has had cancer, more than 20 dentists, surgeons, cancer specialists, and other professionals have been involved in her treatment. This reflects the complex nature of such cases and the fact that decisions about treatment had to be discussed thoroughly by teams of professionals. All treatment options and their consequences were carefully explained to the patient and her husband.

In this case, the treatment teams also faced a number of psychological problems within the patient's family. Having been a model in her twenties, the patient found it difficult to come to terms with the normal consequences of aging. She and her husband also were unable to accept that facial cancer and the necessary life-saving surgery results in facial disfigurement. In addition, her adopted teenage son died under tragic circumstances during the period of her cancer treatment, which added to the family's psychological distress during this time.

Patient History

This patient was first referred to Sahlgren's Hospital in Gothenburg, Sweden, in 1982 at the age of 48. An adenoid cystic cancer of her left parotid gland was diagnosed, and during that year three separate operations were performed to remove the tumor. At this point, none of the procedures were radical in nature.

However, the patient had said that she was "very concerned" about her facial expressions and a face-lift was subsequently carried out in 1984. Having been a fashion model, and still carrying out some fashion work even in her late 40s, she believed that an attractive appearance was of paramount importance.

Following a tooth extraction in 1987, it was discovered that the cancer had returned. This time, however, the patient would have to be treated with more radical procedures.

Both the patient and her spouse were fully informed of the nature and consequences of the procedure to be carried out. In July, the surgeon performed a modified Ferguson approach to gain access to the tumor site. This involved an incision in the upper lip and followed the contour of the nose. The resultant cheek flap was then reflected. A partial maxillectomy on the left side of the face was performed. It was not possible, however, to remove all of the tumor growth, which had spread further into the jaw and palate. Following discussions with other cancer specialists, it was decided that rather than perform even more radical surgery, the best option was radiation therapy.

Radiation therapy treatment was begun the next month but had to be halted following a severe reaction by the patient—her upper lip and left cheek had become swollen. Within one month of ceasing the radiation therapy, the patient's condition improved, although her ability to open her mouth was limited. As a consequence, she was unable to use a prosthetic obturator. To close the open passage between the oral and nasal cavities, the patient had to place a piece of cotton wool into the maxillary defect (Fig 8-1).

As a consequence, frequent and increasingly severe infections in original mucosa and grafted skin covering the remaining bone surfaces in the walls of the maxillary defect occurred. In 1989 an infection in her operated left side proved difficult to control despite various antibiotic treatments.

Increasingly, the patient had become dependent on a variety of analgesics, including Morphiate. In 1990, she prepared to undertake detoxification treatment to free herself of the addiction.

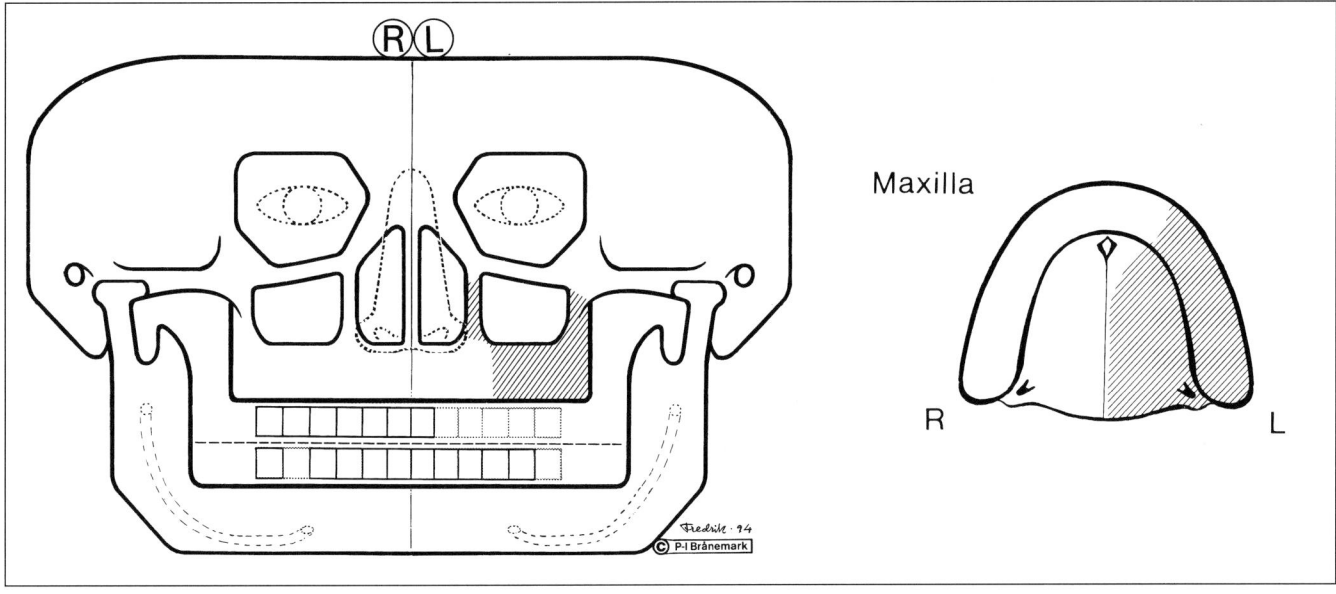

Fig 8-1 Delineation of the maxillary defect.

Rehabilitation

Not until September 1990, with 8 years' treatment history and a variety of physical, psychological, and family problems present, was she referred for consultation concerning possibilities to improve her oral rehabilitation, particularly to occlude the communication between oral and nasal cavities, but primarily to allow her to open her mouth to control the serious recurrent mucosal infections.

One of the contraindications to craniofacial rehabilitation is the patient's belief that such treatment can fully restore appearance to that prior to radical cancer therapy. A psychiatrist identified such a problem in this patient. Despite the strong contraindications from a psychological point of view, including unreasonable expectations of the rehabilitation treatment, it was felt that the patient could benefit from such treatment for three main reasons: it would enable the patient to open her mouth wider; to reduce the localized tissue pain; and to close the defect inside the mouth between the oral and nasal cavities using a bone-anchored obturator to eliminate the need for cotton wool.

After undergoing hyperbaric oxygen treatment, the patient underwent surgery in March 1992. Several procedures were performed. First was an operation on the temporomandibular joint, after which the mouth opening could be increased to about 26 mm, compared with only a few millimeters previously. Three fixtures were then inserted in the remaining mesial maxillary base to the left, including a bone graft from the hip. One fixture was also installed in the base of the left zygomatic arch.

A second period of hyperbaric oxygen treatment was carried out, and the patient also received special training to improve her ability to open her mouth further. Then, in June 1993, the patient underwent a second operation for the attachment of abutments and the excision of a mucosal polyp. Abutments were attached to three fixtures, while one fixture was removed due to lack of integration in grafted bone. The mucous membrane was carefully realigned.

After healing of soft tissues, adjustment and fitting of an obturator prosthesis and a bar construction was performed. Over the following weeks, small adjustments were made to the bar and prosthesis to allow comfortable function. While the patient expressed satisfaction with her prosthesis, she was not content with the contraction of her left upper cheek. It was believed that tissue shrinkage was continuing and that a nonangulated abutment on the zygomatic fixture should be replaced by an angulated one. As a result, the bar was taken off and the distal segment reduced. Only two front fixtures were used subsequently for the now-shortened bar construction.

Because the two frontal fixtures provided adequate stability for the obturator, it was decided to leave the fixture in the zygomatic arch without an abutment, covered by mucosa, but available for connection if the frontal fixtures and the patient's remaining teeth should be lost.

Three weeks later, the patient complained that the left corner of her mouth was still retracted, that she had pain in her left jaw, and that she had vision difficulties in her left eye.

In the following week, the patient suffered a dislocation in her right jaw, which meant that she could not use her upper prosthesis for fear of new dislocation. She was also unable to train her bite, and her ability to open her mouth was further reduced. This also meant that she could not insert her obturator prosthesis. Insertion became possible following adjustments to the prosthesis, and retention was improved as well.

The patient was provided with capsplints (metal caps placed over the teeth) in the upper and lower jaw, which enabled her to continue vigorous manual opening exercises with the aid of increasing numbers of wooden spatulas according to the Ridell procedure, with a maximum of 16 spatulas. This resulted in an opening of 23 mm some few weeks' postoperatively.

DIFFICULTIES

Throughout her illness, the patient had suffered considerably at various periods because of difficult-to-control problems. At this point, the patient felt that not everything had been done to improve her appearance.

In mid-1993, it was suspected that certain changes in the left orbit were due to a malignant process, but at that time it was believed that tumor growth was slow. Neither the patient or her husband, however, would acknowledge the possibility of this new tumor growth. Further, the patient would not undergo fine needle biopsy to verify the diagnosis, or radiation therapy, on the grounds that it would have meant the loss of vision in her left eye.

She was also upset about her appearance, despite the restoration of function and closure of the defect internally. Her radiation therapy specialist feared a suicide attempt if some consideration of plastic surgery was not made. For that reason, a plastic surgeon at Harvard Medical School was asked to consider the possibilities of correction using plastic surgery techniques. He pointed out that there was the danger that a tumor was still present. He felt that before any reconstruction using plastic surgery was considered, the existence of the tumor should be confirmed and treated.

This surgeon believed that the patient was unwilling to acknowledge the nature of her illness. This resulted in her belief that all those involved in her treatment had made errors. Furthermore, the patient had complained that her facial damage was due to incompetence of those treating her, rather than the consequence of the cancer or the oncologic treatment procedures, and *threatened legal action.*

The surgeon felt that this patient needed to come to terms with the reality of her medical condition and accept the treatment regimen. He acknowledged that her problem was, anatomically and biologically, difficult to resolve. However, this, coupled with the underlying psychiatric condition, had made the treatment situation difficult to resolve, and it remained a deep concern for all those involved in treating this patient.

Discussion

This case description illustrates well the complex problems that can arise as a result of reconstructive surgery following cancer treatment in the facial region. The fundamental problem is the patient's disease and the defects that arise as a result of cancer surgery and radiation therapy. There is a considerable risk that the patient will both deny the cancer and have unrealistic expectations of the treatment results.

For the patient to be helped by reconstructive treatment, he or she must completely accept the situation, the prognosis, and the natural course of events. Further, the patient must understand and accept that it is not possible to *completely* restore function or features cosmetically either with implant surgery or any other type of treatment. With this attitude, a patient can feel that even a modest functional improvement is a dramatic change.

In the case described, comprehensive information and treatment options for both the cancer and implant surgery along with consequence of such treatment were given. Despite this, the patient had unrealistic expectations of complete restoration to her former state, cosmetically and functionally. When these expectations were not realized, she viewed the results as treatment errors.

All treatment aims to help the patient. It is thus a difficult balance with this type of patient, who despite the obvious improvement in function believes that she has been wrongly treated or that insufficient treatment has been performed. It is tempting for the responsible treatment professional to do the least possible or nothing at all. (These and similar issues were considered in an editorial, "A Trial of Disputation," in Lancet Vol 343, No. 8888, 1994.

A prerequisite for successful treatment is a relationship of trust between doctor and patient. This can be achieved only if the treating doctor is prepared to do all that is realistic and the patient accepts this. Of course, the anaplastologist may be particularly at risk of exposure to unrealistic expectations from the patient for a return to previous anatomy or even to supranormal appearance.

To try to avoid disturbances in the relation between patient and health-care providers, it might be appropriate, after reviewing the suggested treatment protocol verbally, to formalize the treatment plan in the form of a contract between the patient and those involved in the treatment. This contract would give a detailed description of the treatment goals with different treatment phases and their associated risks. After a suitable time in which to consider and clear up any uncertainties in the contract's contents, the patient should then sign a document that he or she has decided to be treated in a particular way, that he or she has been informed in detail about the situation, and that he or she accepts not only the treatment plan but also any risks and side effects.

While not a legally binding contract, such a document provides a foundation for treatment, ensuring that the patient is well informed and has thought through his or her decision. A situation in which subsequent rehabilitation work takes place with unrealistic expectations is thus avoided.

Concluding Remarks

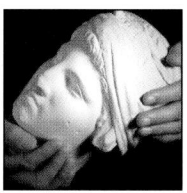

Per-Ingvar Brånemark

PROSTHETIC REHABILITATION of craniomaxillofacial defects based on osseointegration requires considerable surgical and particularly anaplastologic skill to achieve an acceptable level of function and esthetics. Treatment planning is crucial, and the participation of an anaplastologist in the presurgical selection of optimum position and direction of anchoring elements, as well as in the adaptation of a soft-tissue margin to accommodate the prosthesis, is essential for the final result. These basic facts are clearly illustrated by the two separate sections of this book.

The important interaction between health-care providers and patients is another element affecting the acceptance of prosthetic substitution for lost anatomic structures. Such patients require careful attention to their individual anatomic and mental conditions. Sufficient time spent on these issues prior to treatment is a prerequisite for predictable long-term rehabilitation.

The first section of this book clearly demonstrates that excellent prosthetic substitution can be provided even in complicated cases. It is, however, also important to emphasize the need for continued development, not only in anaplastologic methods but also in materials, to make prostheses last longer and feel and look more natural, and to reduce the overall treatment costs by simplifying individualized manufacturing techniques.

The preparation of this book has been a most gratifying experience in learning how individual anaplastologists have achieved a remarkable level of success in their basically manual production of substitutes for lost human anatomic structures.